CU00794172

Self-Assessment Colour Review of

Small Animal Dermatology

Karen A. Moriello DVM DACVD
Department of Medical Sciences
School of Veterinary Medicine
University of Wisconsin-Madison
Wisconsin, USA

ROYAL CANIN

This book is a gift to you from Royal Canin – supporting the global
veterinary community through research driven by knowledge,
respect, passion for cats and dogs and a spirit of innovation.

MANSON PUBLISHING/THE VETERINARY PRESS

Dedication
To Mark and Ethan
Thanks TEAM!
OSU!

Acknowledgements

Any clinical text is partly the creation of the author and partly the creation of other 'unnamed contributors' who have influenced the author either directly, or indirectly.

With that in mind, I would like to thank the following people: Drs. Richard Halliwell, Gail Kunkle, and Valerie Fadok, my mentors, colleagues, and friends. Drs. Danny Scott, Bill Miller, and Craig Griffin, who are currently entrusted with keeping the 'bible' of veterinary dermatology current and updated. This book was an invaluable aid in preparation of this text. And last, but not least, Dr. Douglas J. DeBoer, my friend and colleague since we joined the faculty at the University of Wisconsin in 1986.

I would also like to thank the following people for reviewing and editing this text: Dr. Lane Hansen (Class of 2003); Dr. Angela Kadwig (Class of 2003); Dr Jesse Sondel (Class of 2003); Dr. Michele Turek, DACVO; Dr. Melissa Wallace, DACVIM; Dr. Erin Dickerson.

A CIP catalogue record for this book is available from the British Library.

For full details of all Manson Publishing Ltd titles please write to:
Manson Publishing Ltd, 73 Corringham Road, London NW11 7DL, UK.

Tel: +44(0)20 8905 5150
Fax: +44(0)20 8201 9233

Email: manson@mansonpublishing.com
Website: www.manson-publishing.co.uk

Commissioning editor: Jill Northcott
Project manager: Paul Bennett
Copy editor: Ruth Maxwell
Page layout: Initial Typesetting Services
Colour reproduction: Tenon & Polert Colour Scanning Ltd, Hong Kong
Printed in China by New Era Printing Company Ltd

Preface

This book is a general review of veterinary dermatology in a case-based format. The book reviews the most common skin diseases encountered in clinical practice. I have tried hard to include the most common skin diseases, and a few obscure ones that a clinician will encounter from time to time. It is not within the scope of this book to review every skin disease in detail. If more information is needed on a particular disease or some aspect of it, the reader is referred to the latest edition of the *Textbook of Small Animal Dermatology* (DW Scott, WH Miller, C Griffin [eds]. WB Saunders, Philadelphia).

Karen A. Moriello

Picture acknowledgements

Picture acknowledgements in veterinary dermatology can be difficult to credit. This is because veterinary dermatologists swap slides like collectors swap baseball trading cards. In the process of many 'swaps' the original owner of the slide is often lost because slides are 'gifted' from one person to another. Over the last 20 years I have been the beneficiary of many 'slide gifts' from my mentors, resident mates, and colleagues. I have tried to credit the original owner of the slide or institution where the slide originated, if possible. I apologize if someone recognizes a slide of theirs and they were not credited. In those cases, I hope the original clinician of record is pleased with the way in which the illustration was used, and I would like to thank them now.

The cases in this book originate in one way or another from the teaching material and/or dermatology training programs. I would specifically like to acknowledge the following institutions: The School of Veterinary Medicine, University of Wisconsin-Madison, Madison Wisconsin, USA. The School of Veterinary Medicine, University of California-Davis, Davis California, USA. The College of Veterinary Medicine, University of Florida, Gainesville Florida, USA. The School of Veterinary Medicine, University of Pennsylvania, Philadelphia Pennsylvania, USA. The College of Veterinary Medicine, Cornell University, Ithaca New York, USA.

I would like to thank the following people for generously allowing me to use cases from their slide collections: Dr. Douglas J. DeBoer, University of Wisconsin-Madison; Dr. Gail Kunkle, University of Florida; Dr. William Miller, Cornell University; Dr. David Vail, University of Wisconsin-Madison; Dr. Stuart Helfand, University of Wisconsin-Madison; Dr. Michele Turek, University of Wisconsin-Madison.

Broad classification of cases

1 While practicing small animal medicine in a warm subtropical climate, one morning in June a 6-year-old mixed breed dog was examined for the complaint of intense pedal pruritus. Prior to this episode, the dog had no history of previous skin diseases. Except for the feet, which were wet from constant chewing and licking, the dog's skin was otherwise normal. The dorsal and interdigital areas were normal; the dog had chewed most intensely on the plantar surface and at the junction of the pad and haired skin. The feet were swollen, self-traumatized, and in multiple sites the hard cornified pad was missing (1a). The medical record revealed that the client practiced good preventive care (including monthly flea control and monthly heartworm prevention with a product with label claim to prevent intestinal parasites). The dog was walked several times a day, and three or four times a week it visited a local park where it could

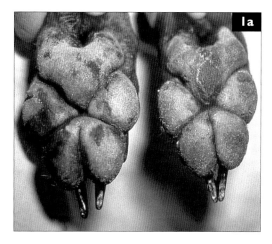

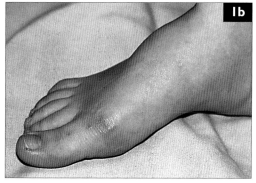

run freely. Incidentally, the owner complained of intensely pruritic feet; she wore sandals to the park (1b).

i. The final diagnosis in this case was 'hookworm dermatitis'. What other differential diagnoses were most likely considered, what dermatological diagnostic tests were probably done at the time of presentation, and what is the general pathogenesis of this disease?

ii. What should the owner be told when she asks why the dog's heartworm medication did not prevent this infestation, and how best should the dog be treated?

iii. The pathogenesis of 'hookworm dermatitis' has been studied with natural and experimental infestations with *Uncinaria stenocephala*. What were those findings, where is this parasite most commonly found, and what host is its reservoir?

I: Answer

1 i. In addition to hookworm dermatitis, *Pelodera* dermatitis, demodicosis, and contact dermatitis were the most likely differential diagnoses. The acute onset of lesions and the lack of a history of previous skin disease made atopic dermatitis unlikely. Skin scrapings were negative in this dog ruling out *Demodex* and *Pelodera*, which are easily found on skin scrapings. In most cases of hookworm dermatitis, skin scrapings are negative. Impression smears and/or cytological scrapings of material from the nail bed and interdigital areas were performed to look for bacterial and/or *Malassezia* yeast infection. The history, clinical findings, and diagnostic testing made the diagnosis of hookworm dermatitis most likely. In hookworm dermatitis, the larvae of *Ancylostoma* or *Uncinaria* are present on grass and in the soil of contaminated areas in the spring and summer, and percutaneously invade the skin of dogs (and people). Intense pruritus can occur if the dog is exposed to large numbers of larva. This is a disease of dogs kenneled on grass or earth runs where sanitation is poor. In dogs, cutaneous lesions are most common with the larvae of *U. stenocephala*.

ii. Heartworm medications do not provide complete protection against hookworm dermatitis because therapeutic concentrations are only present for a short time after the once monthly administration, allowing the dog to be at risk for an infestation. Short-term use of glucocorticoids will alleviate the pruritus. Ivermectin (200 μg/kg PO q24h) has been used to kill migrating larvae. For long-term control, the use of heartworm preventatives should be continued; however, it is most important to keep the dog away from unsanitary areas. This parasitic disease is easily prevented by good sanitation (daily removal of feces) and exercising the dog in a clean area. There is an increasing occurrence of this disease in urban areas where off-leash dog exercise parks have become popular. A fecal examination should be done, and the dog treated for hookworms with an appropriate antihelmintic even though it is receiving a heartworm preventive with claims to prevent intestinal parasites.

iii. Experimental and natural infections with *U. stenocephala* indicate the third stage larvae will readily enter skin in contact with the ground (Matthews, 1981; Scott *et al.*, 2001a). Larvae can be found in contaminated soil and also on dew-laden grass. Infective larvae will enter the skin via hair follicles or areas of desquamation. The most common sites of penetration are at areas of normal 'wear and tear': bony prominences of elbows, hocks, margins of the footpads and haired skin, nail beds, and the ischial tuberosities. Larvae enter the skin at the stratum corneum. They push against the rigid epidermal cells and move forward in an undulating motion. The larvae move about 2–3 mm a day in the skin following paths of least resistance. The dermis does not seem to hinder their progress, and after larvae pass through the tissues, the cells reunite leaving little evidence of their presence. Histological examination of infested tissue is remarkably similar to 'hypersensitivity reactions'. Tracks of larvae may be found, but larvae themselves are rare. *Ancylostoma* spp. is the canine hookworm parasite most commonly found in subtropical or tropical regions of the world. *U. stenocephala* is more commonly found in cooler climates, where it is primarily a fox parasite.

2 A 5-year-old male Norwegian elkhound dog with generalized confluent dermal masses is shown (2). The tumors are firm to fluctuant, well-circumscribed, dermal to subcutaneous masses varying in size from 0.5–>5.0 cm. Some of the lesions have visible pores opening onto the surface of the skin; the pores are filled with cutaneous plugs. The dog is otherwise healthy.

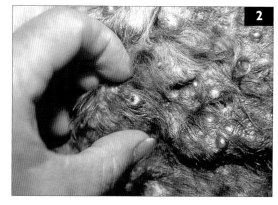

i. What is the most likely diagnosis, what treatment options are available, and what is the prognosis?
ii. What is this the origin of these tumors?
iii. If this tumor were aspirated, what would a cytological examination be expected to find?

3 The local fire department rescued an adult cat from the attic of a house on fire. The heat was so intense the floor vinyl beneath the cat's hind paws melted and adhered to his fur. The firemen cut the vinyl floor from beneath the cat and brought the cat to the veterinary clinic with its paws adhered to the flooring. Under anesthesia, the melted floor vinyl was removed from the cat's fur. The cat's paws were burned (3). The skin beneath the wounds was erythematous and bled during the debridement.

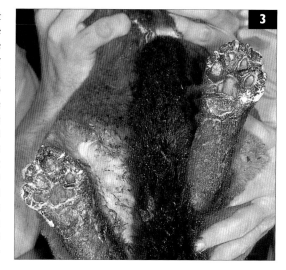

i. Is this a partial or full thickness burn?
ii. How should this patient's burns be managed?
iii. What is erythema ab igne?

2, 3: Answers

2 i. Keratoacanthoma (also called an intracutaneous cornifying epithelioma). This is a benign neoplasm that can be solitary or multiple. Norwegian elkhound and keeshond dogs are predisposed to the generalized form. Single lesions can be confused with cutaneous horns or epidermal cysts because they look similar. These lesions are differentiated by histological examination of tissue. Solitary keratoacanthomas can be treated by surgical excision, cryotherapy, electrotherapy, and observation without treatment. Multiple lesions are usually too numerous for surgical excision. Oral retinoids (isotretinoin 1–3 mg/kg PO q24h) have been successful in the treatment of multiple keratoacanthomas in some dogs. Treatment responses may take up to 3 months and, if effective, need life-long administration. Considered benign proliferations of skin epithelium, these lesions are benign, non-invasive, and do not metastasize. Dogs with generalized lesions have a strong tendency to develop new tumors at other sites. The generalized form is believed to have a hereditary basis in dogs.

ii. These tumors originate from the superficial epithelium between hair follicles although some may originate from adnexa.

iii. Cytologically, these tumors are characterized by keratin debris, rafts of keratinocytes, keratin bars, cholesterol crystals, and inflammatory cells if the mass has ruptured. These tumors can be difficult to differentiate from inclusion cysts.

3 i. This is a partial thickness burn. These burns involve the epidermis and superficial dermis. In full thickness burns, there is complete destruction of the epidermis, dermis, skin glands, and hair follicles.

ii. The wounds should be cleaned and debrided as needed. Daily hydrotherapy 2–3 times a day will help remove dead tissue and exudates. Because the hair coat of many patients obscures the skin, the full extent of this cat's burns may not be visible for up to 72 hours. The fluid and electrolyte balance must also be monitored. This cat's paws were treated daily with silver sulfadiazine ointment and bandages changed twice daily. The paws healed, and the cat functioned normally. Patients caught in house fires may have significant heat and/or smoke damage to their respiratory tract.

iii. Erythema ab igne, also called chronic moderate heat dermatitis, is an erythematous reticular macular dermatitis that occurs at the site of repeated exposure to moderate heat (Walder and Hargis, 2002). It is a type of a chronic burn. In animals, there is erythema and hyperpigmentation at the site, and alopecia is common. Lesions may have an irregular, linear appearance. The most common sources of 'moderate heat' that small animals may encounter include open fires, heat lamps, electric blankets, electric heating pads, hot water bottles, and steam radiators. It is also observed in dogs and cats that sleep on sun-heated driveways or on sun-heated concrete.

4 A circular crusted lesion was found on the abdomen of a dog (4). The owner reports the lesion was a small red bump yesterday, and today there is this crusted lesion.

i. What are these lesions called?

ii. What other skin disease(s) can this lesion be mistaken for clinically?

iii. What is superficial spreading pyoderma?

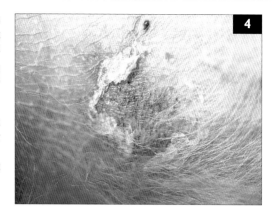

5 The owners of an adult Labrador retriever dog with a history of chronic 'nasal dermatitis' presented the dog for an emergency examination. Until now, the owners had refused all recommendations for diagnostic testing to determine the cause of the nasal crusting shown (5). The crusting has been present for almost 2 years, and it did not seem to be problematic to the dog. The dog is presented today with the complaint of epistaxis. Closer questioning of the owners

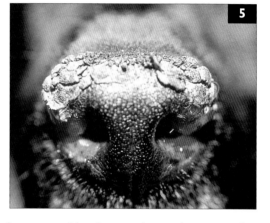

reveals the epistaxis is a recent development and has happened on at least two other occasions. On physical examination, the dog is normal except for the skin. There are no signs of petechial hemorrhage on any of the mucous membranes. Dermatological examination reveals thick adherent crusting on the dorsum of the nose and bilateral ulceration of the nares. The blood appears to be coming from these ulcerative areas. There was no exposure to rodenticides.

i. What are the differential diagnoses? What must also be ruled out?

ii. What diagnostic tests should be performed on this patient?

iii. If this patient had presented for the problem of chronic nasal crusting without any evidence of erosions and ulcerations of the nares, what benign hereditary disease should be considered?

4 i. This lesion is called an epidermal collarette, and is representative of a superficial bacterial pyoderma. It results from the rupture of an intact pustule. After the pustule ruptures, a crust develops and spreads in a circular fashion creating a 'collar of crust'. There may or may not be a ring of erythema at the margin. As the lesion heals, the center often becomes hyperpigmented.

ii. Epidermal collarettes are commonly misidentified as 'ringworm lesions' or dermatophytosis. Skin scrapings should be done to rule out demodicosis. If there are other dermatological signs consistent with dermatophytosis, a fungal culture should be performed. Pending fungal culture, the patient is best treated with a minimum of a 21 day course of antibiotics; treatment should continue for 1 week past clinical cure. If skin scrapings and fungal cultures are negative and the patient does not respond to appropriate antibiotic therapy, a skin biopsy is indicated to rule out other rare causes of these lesions (e.g. PF).

iii. Superficial spreading pyoderma is a bacterial pyoderma characterized by large epidermal collarettes with an erythematous, mild exudative/crusted leading edge. What is unique about this clinical form of superficial pyoderma is the lack of pustules; lesions are extensive and pustules are conspicuously absent. In the author's experience this form of bacterial pyoderma is often seen in longhaired dogs, especially collie and Shetland sheepdogs, and lesions are common on the trunk.

5 i. The recurrent epistaxis may be due to the skin disease; however, an underlying coagulopathy must be ruled out. The symmetrical nature of the ulcerative nares and nasal crusting is most consistent with lupus erythematosus, pemphigus erythematosus or foliaceus (early onset), epitheliotrophic lymphoma, drug reaction, and contact dermatitis.

ii. A coagulopathogy should be ruled out before obtaining skin biopsy specimens of the depigmented area of the nares and the crusted planum nasale. In this case, a mucosal bleeding time was normal, as was a platelet count. After determining the dog did not have a coagulopathy, skin biopsies were obtained under general anesthesia. Unlike other skin diseases, the best lesions to sample are 'older' lesions. In this case, a biopsy was obtained from the crusted and depigmented areas. To avoid excessive hemorrhage, biopsy specimens should not be taken from the center of the nose as there is a large vessel in this area.

This was a case of cutaneous lupus erythematosus. This disease can be treated with a variety of drugs including glucocorticoids, Vitamin E, tetracycline and niacinamide, and other immunosuppressive anti-inflammatory drugs.

iii. Hereditary nasal parakeratosis of Labrador retriever dogs.

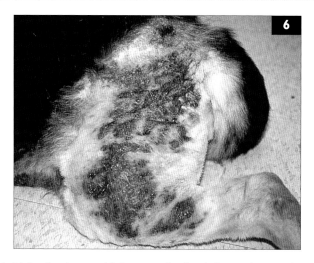

6 The lateral thigh of a 4-year-old German shepherd dog is shown after the hair coat was clipped (6). The dog was presented because of fever, depression, lameness, and 'hard skin'. Upon examination, the 'hard skin' was found to be diffuse exudation matting the hair coat. The skin was painful to the dog.
i. What is the clinical term for these lesions, and what diagnostics should be performed?
ii. What is the significance of the breed of the dog in this case?
iii. What immunological abnormalities have been found in German shepherd dogs with this disease?

7 The lateral abdomen of a 5-year-old English bulldog is shown. The owners were presenting the dog for evaluation of a solitary, well-circumscribed, raised lesion (7). The lesion was firm on palpation and was observed to swell and become edematous after manipulation. What skin tumor is most likely to exhibit this behavior?

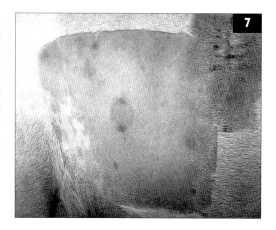

6 i. Deep pyoderma. The hallmarks of deep pyoderma are pain, fever, matting of the hair coat, blood and pus exuding from the lesion, and/or necrosis of tissue. Skin scrapings should be done to rule out demodicosis, the most common cause of deep bacterial pyoderma in the dog. Impression smears should be taken to look for bacterial, fungal, or other infectious agents. It is important to note the presence of cocci, rods, and/or a mixed infection as this may impact initial treatment recommendations pending culture and sensitivity. The presence of large numbers of extracellular bacteria *not* being engulfed by neutrophils suggests a defect in the skin immune system. This can also be observed in dogs that have received glucocorticoid therapy. Finally, this could suggest bacterial overgrowth and be of no significance to the dog.

In the author's experience, however, impression smears with this pattern are almost never of 'no significance to the patient'. Bacterial overgrowth is always due to some underlying change in the skin's environment. Bacterial culture and sensitivity of the exudates should be done, especially if the dog has received previous antibiotic therapy or glucocorticoids, and/or a mixed population of bacteria on cytological examination of exudates is confirmed. This is a cost effective diagnostic test because resolution of the infection will require 4–12 weeks of antibiotics. Skin biopsy should also be performed to rule out other causes of deep pyoderma, such as superficial or deep fungal infections.

ii. This is a case of GSDP. This syndrome is poorly understood and the cause is unknown. It has been proposed to be caused by a defect in the skin immune system of certain breeding lines of German shepherd dogs, and there is often a familial history of severe deep pyoderma. This is a disease of middle-aged dogs. Lesions can occur anywhere but are most common on the rump, dorsal back, ventral abdomen, and lateral thighs. All above-mentioned diagnostic tests are indicated, as well as a thyroid function test. Treatment involves clipping of the hair coat, whirlpool soaks in antibacterial solutions (e.g. chlorhexidine), and long courses of antibiotics. Fluoroquinolone antibiotics may be especially useful because they are concentrated in inflammatory cells and are effective in the presence of exudates, granulation tissue, and fibrosis. Incomplete response to antibiotic therapy and/or frequent relapses are common. Neutering and removal from the breeding program of affected dogs and their offspring are suggested.

iii. A small number of affected dogs were studied and found to have increased numbers of CD8+ and decreased numbers of CD4+ and CD21+ lymphocytes, in addition to low serum IgA concentrations. Skin biopsies from affected dogs showed a markedly lower number of lymphocytes in the skin than in cases from other breeds (Scott *et al.*, 2001b).

7 MCT. Canine MCT may enlarge after manipulation due to degranulation of mast cells.

8 This adult dog was presented with lameness and foot chewing. Physical examination revealed a nonweight-bearing lameness of the right foreleg. The dog was placed in lateral recumbency, and an orthopedic examination was done to try to localize the pain. The digits were examined; large numbers of foreign objects were found interdigitally and on the plantar surface of the paw (8).

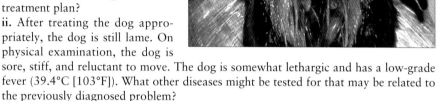

i. What is the diagnosis and treatment plan?
ii. After treating the dog appropriately, the dog is still lame. On physical examination, the dog is sore, stiff, and reluctant to move. The dog is somewhat lethargic and has a low-grade fever (39.4°C [103°F]). What other diseases might be tested for that may be related to the previously diagnosed problem?
iii. What are the most common zoonotic diseases transmitted by this parasite, and how are owners at risk for contracting these diseases?

9 This cat was presented for the complaint of hair loss and overgrooming in the caudal thigh region (9). The owner reports that the cat often 'jumps up, growls, and starts biting and grooming itself'. Flea combing was negative for fleas or flea feces. A clinical diagnosis of FAD was made, and the cat's overgrooming, hair loss, and odd behavior all resolved when the cat was treated with a monthly spot-on flea control product. The owner wants to know how this can be a flea problem when fleas were not found on examination. What should she be told?

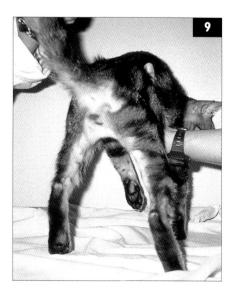

8 i. Severe interdigital tick infestation. Ticks are commonly found on paws between the toes. In this patient, large numbers of ticks were present causing lameness. Dogs with heavy infestations should be treated with a fipronil- or permethrin-based spray. Topical sponge-on dips labeled for fleas and ticks can be used, and repeat applications are needed for maximum efficacy. Single ticks can be removed manually using a metal tick remover or forceps. Because of the risk of tick borne diseases, injury to the dog, and incomplete removal of the tick's head, owners should be cautioned against manual detachment of the ticks. In this case, manual removal of the ticks would be impossible, even if the dog was heavily sedated or anesthetized. It is more practical, humane, and safe to use a parasiticidal drug to kill the ticks. The owner should be cautioned that there might be detached, engorged ticks present around the home, kennel, on the dog, or on other dogs in the home. The home may need to be treated to prevent a tick infestation. Finally, a recommendation should be made for prevention of future tick infestations. Fipronil, amitraz-impregnated collars, and selamectin (for *Dermacentor variabilis*) can be used to prevent tick infestations.

ii. Given the dog's recent severe tick infestation, serious consideration must be given to a possible tick borne infection that can cause polyarthritis. Serum titers for ehrlichiosis, *Rickettsia* (Rocky Mountain spotted fever), and borreliosis (Lyme's disease) would be indicated in this patient. Diagnosis is often difficult because many dogs will have positive antibody titers for these diseases. In many instances, a presumptive 'definitive diagnosis' is made after response to antibiotic therapy (e.g. doxycycline).

iii. The definition of a zoonotic disease is one that is shared by people and pets, not just transmitted from people to animals. The most common tick borne zoonoses are *Rickettsia rickettsia* (Rocky Mountain spotted fever), *Ehrlichia* spp., *Coxiella burnetii* (Q-fever), *Borrelia burgdorferia* (Lyme disease), and *Bartonella henselae* (CSD).

There are three major ways that people are at risk for contracting a tick borne disease. First, direct exposure to an infected tick that bites, attaches, and transmits the disease. Second, the pet can mechanically transport unattached ticks into the home, etc. where they crawl around and find a human host. Third, contact with infected hemolymph from the tick can transmit infective organisms. This is most likely to occur when owners manually remove ticks from pets.

9 FAD is a hypersensitivity reaction. The irritation is so severe that the host (dog or cat) bites and chews at the area where the bite occurred and seems to 'hunt the fleas down' in their hair coat. This is often seen as nibbling, corncob biting, or over-grooming. Cats are particularly vigilant about grooming their coat if they become infested with fleas.

10 A 2-year-old hound dog cross from Florida was presented for examination of nonhealing wounds on the skin. The dog and owner had traveled extensively in the USA, especially in the mid-western region. The dog had been used for duck and raccoon hunting 4–6 months before the lesions were first noted. The lesions drained a thick purulent exudate and were moderately painful but cool to the touch. On physical examination there was generalized lymphadenopathy and draining lymph nodes (10), weight loss, and cough, but ocular examination was normal. The dog was febrile and depressed.

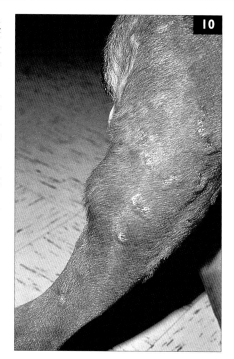

i. What are the differential diagnoses?
ii. What is the most cost effective diagnostic approach using only in-house diagnostic tests?
iii. Assuming the cause of the lesion and lymphadenopathy has not been identified, what other diagnostic tests should be performed?

11 An impression smear of the exudates of the dog in 10 is shown (11).

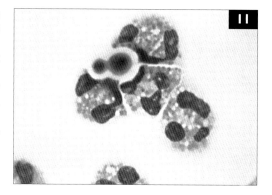

i. What is the diagnosis, and what are the treatment options?
ii. How did the dog most likely contract this organism? Is this a zoonosis?
iii. What is the prognosis for this disease?

10 i. The dog's dermatological problem is a nonhealing wound. The differential diagnoses for nonhealing wounds in dogs are legion and include deep bacterial infections, intermediate mycoses, deep mycoses, and neoplasia. The concurrent signs of systemic illness (fever, depression, weight loss, cough, and lymphadenopathy) suggest that the skin lesions are secondary to an underlying systemic illness such as infection or neoplasia.

ii. The most cost effective diagnostic tests are skin scrapings to rule out demodicosis; impression smears to look for infectious agents; lymph node aspirate to determine if the lymphadenopathy is reactive, neoplastic, or infectious; and thoracic radiographs. The primary goal of these initial diagnostic tests is establish the cause of the illness. Additional diagnostic tests such as laboratory work (including complete blood count) can be done to assess the dog's overall health once a diagnosis has been made.

iii. Skin biopsies, lung aspirates, and serum titers for deep fungal organisms.

11 i. Canine blastomycosis. Note the septic inflammation and the broad-based, thick-walled, budding yeast. The treatment of choice is itraconazole. It is more effective than ketoconazole and is less toxic than the previous treatment of choice, amphotericin B. The dog should be treated with 5 mg/kg PO q24h for at least 60 days past clinical cure. It is important to note that treatment will require months of therapy.

ii. Blastomycosis is a dimorphic fungus. It is a soil saprophyte, and it transforms into its yeast form in tissues at body temperature. The organism requires a special environmental niche to survive. Where outbreaks of the disease have been investigated, the common factor is sandy, acid wetland areas. Dogs used for duck and raccoon hunting are at greater risk, possibly because the organism is common near waterways in the midwest, especially near beaver dams. The dams create wetlands and marshes that are ideal duck habitat. The mode of infection is via inhalation, and dogs are much more susceptible to the disease than people.

The disease is of limited zoonotic concern as most cases of animal-to-human transmission have occurred due to traumatic inoculation. When owners and dogs contract the disease, it is almost always because both were exposed to the same environmental source.

iii. In general, the prognosis for dogs is good. The two most important prognostic indicators are whether there is brain involvement and severity of lung disease. Dogs with brain involvement usually die. The severity of lung infiltrates may worsen within the first few days of therapy, most likely due to the inflammation. Approximately 50% of dogs with severe lung involvement die as a result of respiratory failure within the first 7 days of treatment.

12 A 5-year-old West Highland white terrier with primary seborrhea is presented for examination for the complaint of intense pruritus of 4 weeks' duration. The diagnosis of primary seborrhea was made several years ago, and the symptoms managed successfully with aggressive shampoo therapy. In the past, pruritus has not been a major dermatological problem for this dog. The owner reported that the pruritus began shortly after the dog was boarded for 3 weeks. Skin scrapings were negative for *Demodex* mites, and no fleas were found on flea combing; the dog receives monthly spot-on flea control. There was no obvious evidence of pyoderma (e.g. pustules, crusts). It is suspected that the dog contracted scabies while at the boarding kennel and is treated with ivermectin every 2 weeks for three treatments. Six weeks after the initial examination, the owner returns with the dog and complains that the pruritus is worse, and the

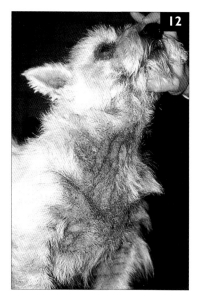

dog's skin is severely seborrheic, malodorous, greasy, and erythematous (12). Impression smears are collected from the neck, face, and nail beds. The exudate from the cracks and crevices of the skin is very oily. The slides are heat fixed and stained.

i. What common microbial infections would an impression smear of this dog's skin be expected to show?
ii. Assuming these two common pathogens are found, how should these combined infections be treated?
iii. What is the proposed relationship between these two organisms?

13 A pair of 8-week-old Labrador retriever puppies is shown (13). Both dogs were born with a normal hair coat, but over the last several weeks one of the puppies has lost its hair coat. Dermatological examination revealed thinning of the hair coat on the puppy's forehead and complete loss of the hair coat on the ventrum.

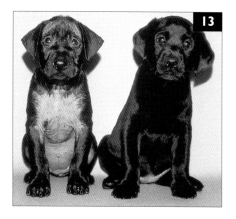

i. What is this condition called?
ii. What would a skin biopsy be expected to show?
iii. What other ectodermal defect is often present in animals with this disorder?

12, 13: Answers

12 i. Concurrent staphylococcal and yeast infections are very common in pruritic patients, especially dogs with atopy and/or seborrhea. *Malassezia* spp. are commonly found on impression smears of the skin, cytological preparations of nail bed debris, and from the scrape preparations of debris from the cracks and crevices of the skin folds. Dogs with disorders of keratinization or those that are predisposed to inflammatory skin diseases commonly develop overcolonization of the skin with bacteria and yeast.

ii. Assuming both are present in this patient, a minimum of 30 days of concurrent treatment for both the bacterial and yeast infection is required. There are two aspects of treatment in any patient with a concurrent bacterial and yeast pyoderma. First, there is the immediate treatment of the yeast dermatitis. One approach is to treat these infections topically with soaks and bathing with antifungal shampoos that contain miconazole and chlorhexidine, ketoconazole, or selenium disulfide, chlorhexidine alone, or enilconazole. Lime sulfur is an antifungal agent, but there are no reports that it is effective in the treatment of yeast dermatitis. If topical treatment alone is used, it needs to be frequent (3–4 times per week). A second treatment approach is with the use of systemic antifungal agents such as ketoconazole or itraconazole; griseofulvin is not effective against *Malassezia*. In the author's experience, topical therapy alone is ineffective in dogs with severe pruritus due to combined infections. If systemic therapy is used, at least 30 days of treatment with ketoconazole or itraconazole (5–10 mg/kg PO q24h) is recommended, and a 30 day course of oral antibiotics is also necessary. The second aspect of therapy is to determine what triggered the overgrowth of yeast in the first place. Primary *Malassezia* infections are uncommon, and overgrowth of this organism is almost always associated with an underlying pruritic and/or seborrheic disease.

iii. There appears to be a symbiotic relationship between staphylococci and yeast that results in the production of growth factors and a mutually beneficial microenvironment. The clinical evidence supporting this hypothesis is that dogs with mixed populations (bacteria and yeast) fare better clinically when both organisms are treated as compared to only one.

13 i. Congenital hypotrichosis, an ectodermal defect. It has been reported in many breeds of dogs and cats. Affected animals may be born without hair or lose their hair coat over the first 4–6 weeks of their life. The hair loss is symmetrical and typically involves the temporal region, ears, caudal thighs, and ventrum. There is no treatment for this disease.

ii. The typical skin biopsy findings are either a complete absence of hair follicles or hypoplastic hair follicles in significantly decreased numbers.

iii. The other ectodermal defect often present is abnormal dentition.

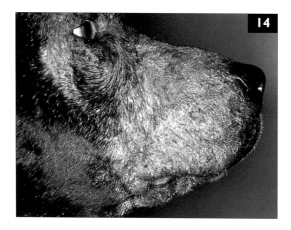

14 A 3-year-old male dog, imported from Portugal, is presented with a history of developing lesions on the face 4 months ago (14). The dog was examined by a veterinarian and reported to be in good health prior to being imported to the USA 1 year ago. The owner reports the dog has lost some weight, is less active, and has mildly itchy scaly skin. On physical examination, marked exfoliative dermatitis is noted on the head, ears, and legs. In addition, there is mild digital hyperkeratosis and paronychia. The dog also has mild lymphadenopathy and splenomegaly. The initial dermatological examination includes skin scrapings (negative for *Demodex* mites), flea combing (negative for fleas and other ectoparasties), a dermatophyte culture (negative), and impression smears of the skin. On the latter, a large numbers of exfoliated keratinocytes, rare cocci, and rare *Malassezia* organisms were noted. A working diagnosis of bacterial and yeast pyoderma is made and a 30 day course of oral antibiotics and topical miconazole shampoo is prescribed. The lymphadenopathy and splenomegaly are worrisome and additional diagnostics are recommended, which the owner declines. At the end of therapy, the dog is no better and has lost another 4 kg (9 lb). The owner reports that the dog is more pruritic.
i. What are the differential diagnoses?
ii. What diagnostic tests are indicated in this patient?
iii. One of the differential diagnoses in this case has two major clinical presentations (cutaneous/mucocutaneous and visceral) and two major geographic distributions (Old World and New World). Briefly describe the two clinical presentations and key differences between the two geographic forms.

15 Fortaz® (ceftazidime) is an injectable drug that is often reformulated by specialty pharmacies to make otic ear drops for the treatment of resistant *Pseudomonas* infections. The concentration of the desired topical solution is 5 mg/ml. Ceftazidime comes in a powder form in a 500 mg vial. How would 100 ml of a 5 mg/ml solution be compounded?

14 i. There are many causes of exfoliative dermatitis; however, the signs of systemic illness in this patient help limit the differential diagnoses to lupus erythematosus, PF, necrolytic migratory erythema, cutaneous lymphoma, and leishmaniasis.

ii. Animals with skin disease and signs of systemic illness require an aggressive work-up. In this patient, a complete blood count, serum chemistry profile, anti-nuclear antibody test, lymph node aspirate, abdominal and thoracic radiographs, and bone marrow aspirate were performed. This was a case of leishmaniasis, and it was diagnosed by finding organisms on skin biopsy, lymph node aspirate, and bone marrow aspirate. This disease is a protozoal infection common in dogs and humans, but it can be seen in cats and other animals. The disease has a worldwide distribution, but it is endemic in the Mediterranean region and Portugal, South and Central America, and in several areas of the USA. It is transmitted by bloodsucking sandflies and causes granulomatous inflammation, immune complex deposition, and related diseases.

The most common skin findings are exfoliative dermatitis with silvery white scales on the face, ears, and legs. Nasodigital hyperkeratosis can occur along with ulcerative dermatitis. Signs of systemic illness are present in about 50% of all cases. This disease is considered incurable and relapses are common. Meglumine antimonate has been used to treat dogs with remission rates over 75%. Other drugs include sodium stibogluconate and allopurinol. This is considered a zoonotic disease, and dogs may be a reservoir of infection for people.

iii. In people, leishmaniasis has two major clinical presentations: cutaneous and mucocutaneous or visceral. In dogs, symptoms usually involve both the skin and viscera.

Old World leishmaniasis in dogs is caused almost exclusively by *L. infantum* or, less commonly, *L. tropica* and is transmitted by sandflies. It is most common in the Mediterranean basin and in Portugal. New World leishmaniasis is endemic in northern and mid-South America, Central America, and is becoming more common in Mexico, the states of Texas and Okalahoma, and the east coast of the USA. The most common species associated with New World disease are *L. mexicana* (complex), *L. braziliensis* (complex), and *L. chagasi*. Over 90% of dogs with overt disease have cutaneous involvement and lymphadenopathy (Slappendel and Ferrer, 1998).

15 Ceftazidine (500 mg vial) can be reconstituted in a 100 ml NaCl 0.9% IV bag to make a solution of 5 mg/ml (500 mg/100 ml = 5 mg/ml ceftazidime [powder volume is insignificant at this volume]).

Note: The author uses ceftazidime for at least 4 weeks of therapy. The reconstituted drug is only stable for 1 week when refrigerated. In order to treat the patient for 4 weeks, the solution is divided into four portions of 25 ml. The three vials of 25 ml for treatment weeks 2, 3, and 4 are kept in the freezer at the patient's home until needed.

16 This 3-year-old indoor-outdoor cat was presented for a second opinion. The owner had been to several veterinarians with the complaint that the cat frequently shook its head and scratched at its ears. Previous diagnostics included ear swabs for mites (negative), cytological examination of ear debris (no organisms found), and flea combing (negative). The owner practiced intermittent flea control. Topical glucocorticoids provided relief, but the cat's symptoms always returned within several days of discontinuing therapy. On this occasion, the cat was presented for severe self-mutilation of the head and neck (16a). Upon examination, severe linear excoriations from the cat's claws were present on the cat's head and neck. The ear canals appeared normal upon otoscopic examination. Ear swabs were negative for mites and microbial organisms. Dermatological examination of the skin revealed erythematous nail beds and interdigital erythema. Skin scrapings of the head and nail bed revealed the organism shown (16b).

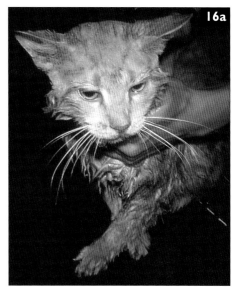

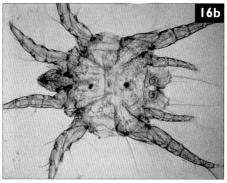

i. What is the diagnosis and treatment?
ii. What is the zoonotic implication of this infestation?
iii. Dogs and cats infested with this organism often have positive intradermal skin test reactions to which mite(s) and why is this clinically significant?

17 What are L-form bacteria?

16 i. The organism is *Otodectes cynotis* (ear mite). Pruritus from ear mites can be due to heavy infestations or, as in this case, due to a hypersensitivity reaction to just a few mites. In some cases of ear mite infestations and/or hypersensitivity reactions, mites may be found in and around the nail beds. In multiple animal situations, systemic treatments may be the treatment of choice, e.g. spot-on fipronil, moxidectin (0.2 mg/kg orally or subcutaneously twice at 10 day intervals), ivermectin (200 µg/kg orally or subcutaneously twice at 10–14 day intervals), ivermectin or milbemycin spot-on treatment for the ears, or selamectin (two treatments at 30 day intervals). In this case, a product containing glucocorticoids would be appropriate to alleviate the intense pruritus. The ears should be cleaned and treated with an appropriate product for at least 4 weeks. Because the mites will migrate on the body, as happened in this case, the cat should be treated with a flea control product to kill migrating ear mites. Failure to do so may result in treatment failure. Concurrent treatment with a topical ear mite treatment and flea control product resulted in resolution of the cat's pruritus.
ii. Although rare, *Otodectes cynotis* is considered a zoonotic disease. Lesions in people have been reported and consist of a papular eruption on the hands and arms (Harwick, 1978). In one anecdotal report (Lopez, 1993), a veterinarian took mite infested ear mite debris and placed it into his own ear, on several occasions. He was able successfully to infest himself with ear mites and reported intense itching. What was most interesting was his observation that the mites were most active at night and could be heard chewing and moving around his ear. This suggests that ear mite preparations would be best applied in the evening. On a more practical level, this also suggests that veterinarians and owners cleaning the ears of pets with ear mite infestations should practice excellent hand washing hygiene post-treatment.
iii. Cats and dogs infested with *Otodectes cynotis* may have positive intradermal skin test reactions to the house dust mites, *Dermatophagoides farinae* and *D. pteronyssinus* (Saridomichelakis, 1999). These reported reactions become negative after the ear mite infestation is eradicated. This is clinically relevant because it would lead to a 'false positive' reaction on an intradermal skin test and a misdiagnosis of atopic dermatitis in a patient with a parasitic infestation. The importance of house dust mites as causes of atopic dermatitis or asthma in cats is increasing, the most likely reason being increased recognition of house dust mites as an allergen. Therefore, ear mite infestations should be ruled out as a possible cause of pruritus before pursuing allergy testing and/or immunotherapy.

17 L-form bacteria are partially cell wall deficient bacteria that resemble *Mycoplasma*. Most reported infections have been associated with abscesses and polyarthropathies.

18 This dog was presented for unilateral periocular inflammation (18). Three weeks ago an infected meibomian gland was lanced and treated with a topical ophthalmic ointment. The meibomian gland infection resolved, but then the periocular area became inflamed, and there was no response to several different antibiotic/ glucocorticoid ophthalmic preparations. There was also no 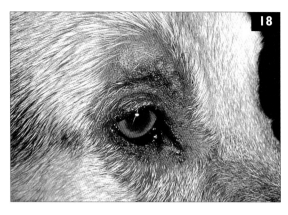 response to a 14 day course of oral antibiotics. Skin scrapings and fungal culture are negative.

i. What is the most likely diagnosis? How could this be confirmed and what is the best course of treatment?

ii. What is a predictable drug reaction versus an unpredictable drug reaction?

iii. List the common cutaneous patterns or conditions associated with adverse drug reactions.

19 A 7-year-old DLH white cat is examined for the complaint of multiple nonhealing wounds on the left hind leg (19), and FNA performed to rule out a mast cell tumor. The FNA is consistent with an epithelial cell tumor. Histological examination of a skin biopsy specimen reveals that it the most common skin tumors of cats.

i. What is it, and what are the most common skin tumors of cats?

ii. What is the prognosis for this tumor?

iii. Is the behavior of this tumor different in dogs?

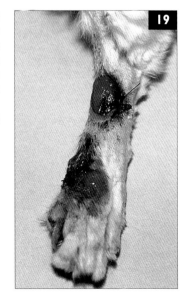

18, 19: Answers

18 i. Localized drug reaction or irritant reaction to one or more of the components in the topical ophthalmic preparations. The unilateral acute nature of the lesions makes allergic disease unlikely. If the lesions were bilateral, allergic disease (atopy or food allergy) would be suspected. The diagnosis can be confirmed via provocative challenge exposure. The best course of treatment is to discontinue all topical therapy to the affected area. If this is a case of a localized drug reaction or an irritant reaction, the lesion should quickly resolve. In this patient, a localized drug reaction was found to topical neomycin sulfate, a drug present in all of the topical preparations used previously. Drug reactions to topical neomycin are very common, particularly in the ears.
ii. Predictable drug reactions are usually dose associated and are related to the pharmacology of the drug. An example of this would be vomiting associated with erythromycin administration. Unpredictable drug reactions are related to an individual animal's immunological response to the drug or to genetic factors associated with the breed. This type of drug reaction could be dose related. An example of this is ivermectin toxicosis in collie dogs. Sensitivity is not uniform in the breed, and toxicity in susceptible individuals can be dose related. Sensitive individuals tolerate the low dose associated with heartworm prevention but not the high dose needed for treatment of parasitic infestations.
iii. Common cutaneous patterns or conditions include urticaria-angioedema, macular-papular eruptions, autoimmune-like disease, erythema multiforme, toxic epidermal necrolysis, pruritus and self-trauma, injection site reactions, allergic contact dermatitis of the ears, vasculitis, fixed drug eruptions, and lichenoid skin disease.

19 i. Basal cell tumor, the most common skin tumor of cats. The most common skin tumors of cats, in descending order, are basal cell tumor, mast cell tumor, squamous cell carcinoma, and fibrosarcoma.
ii. Basal cell tumors commonly occur on the head, neck, thorax, and limbs. Most tumors are solitary, but they can be multiple. They are typically well-encapsulated, well-demarcated, and hairless. The prognosis is good if the tumor is excised completely. Basal cell tumors can be treated by surgical excision, electrosurgery, cryosurgery, or observation without treatment. These tumors have a low incidence of recurrence and tend not to metastasize. In this cat, the tumor was surgically removed, however, wound closure was problematic due to the location. The cat required several surgical procedures to close the defect.
iii. Basal cell tumors in dogs are less common (an estimated 4–12% of all skin tumors), tend to occur in older dogs, and cocker spaniel and poodle breeds seem to have an increased incidence. These tumors have a high mitotic rate for a benign tumor. Rare recurrences have been reported in dogs.

20 A 1-year-old female cocker spaniel dog was presented for head shaking and, more importantly, because it 'stank' (20). Physical examination revealed that the dog's hair coat was greasy, a secondary bacterial pyoderma (characterized by intact pustules and epidermal collarettes) was present, and the footpads were hyperkeratotic. The haircoat on the face, interdigital areas, and ventral neck was matted

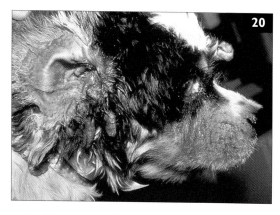

with a malodorous oily yellow material. These lesions have been present since the dog was 4 months of age. The owner would like the skin disease resolved so that the dog could be bred.

i. What should the owner be told?
ii. Which of the retinoids has been most been most effective in the management of disorders of keratinization?
iii. Retinoids have also been used in the treatment of what other diseases?

21 A dog was presented to the surgery department for a femoral fracture. During the case management, the hair over the lumbosacral area was clipped for placement of an epidural catheter for the purpose of pain management. The fracture was repaired and healed without problem. However, the owners are distressed that the hair has not regrown over the lumbosacral area (21). Large breed dogs that have their hair coat clipped over the lumbosacral area may be predisposed to what temporary condition?

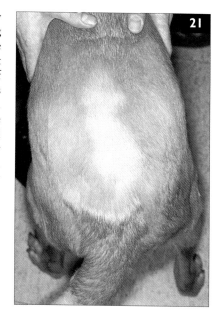

20, 21: Answers

20 i. There are two important points to discuss with the owner. First, the dog has severe seborrhea. The yellowish debris on the face, ears, and hair coat is consistent with primary seborrhea. The history of lesion development when the dog was <4 months of age strongly supports a diagnosis of primary seborrhea of cocker spaniels. This dog's skin disease will be chronic and can be controlled, but not cured. This dog will require life-long therapy for this skin disease that will include special grooming (keeping the hair coat short), frequent bathing (2–3 times a week or more) in medicated shampoos, and treatment of recurrent yeast and bacterial infections.

Second, is that primary seborrhea is an inherited disorder seen in many breeds of dogs, including cocker spaniels. This dog has a particularly severe form of the disease, especially since it started at such a young age. Breeding is not recommended. This patient was evaluated for dermatological and medical causes of primary seborrhea and none were found. A final diagnosis was primary seborrhea along with secondary bacterial and yeast pyoderma. After the secondary infections were resolved, aggressive topical therapy was required to control this primary disorder of keratinization. The dog's hair coat had to be kept short, the ears had to be cleaned daily, and topical otic steroids instilled to control the seborrheic otitis. The owners had to bathe the dog every other day without fail in a tar and sulfur shampoo, benzoyl peroxide shampoo, or an antifungal shampoo, and these topical shampoos were alternated.

ii. The most commonly used retinoids in veterinary dermatology are isotretinoin, etretinate (no longer available), and acitretin. Etretinate was very effective in the treatment of primary idiopathic seborrhea of cocker spaniel and springer spaniel dogs. It was not found to be very effective in West Highland white terrier, basset hound, or collie dogs. This drug is no longer available because tissue residues in people can persist for years, and the drug is very teratogenic. It has been replaced by acitretin, a free radical metabolite of etretinate.

iii. Retinoids have been used to treat ichthyosis, squamous cell carcinoma, keratoacanthomas, sebaceous adentitis, cutaneous lymphoma, and color dilution alopecia.

21 Post-clipping alopecia. This is an idiopathic skin condition characterized by the failure of hair to regrow for as long as 12–24 months after clipping. It is usually seen in large breed dogs with thick hair coats and tends to be localized to the dorsal lumbosacral area. The etiology is unknown, but it is believed to be due to follicular arrest. Additionally, the lack of hair regrowth is due to the long hair cycle of the hairs of this area. It is commonly seen in dogs clipped to remove hair coat mats, but it is observed in dogs clipped for the placement of catheters for epidural anesthesia, myelograms, or surgery.

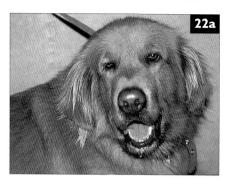
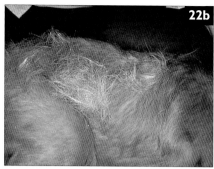

22 A 2-year-old male castrated golden retriever dog was presented for exercise intolerance, weight gain, and excessive shedding (22a). In addition, the owner reported the dog has 'lost his obedience training' and sleeps all of the time. Physical examination reveals an obese dog with a heart rate of 45 beats per minute. The dog's face has a tragic expression. Large clumps of hair are easily epilated from the hair coat (22b).
i. What is the most likely cause of the dog's clinical signs, and what diagnostic tests should be performed?
ii. If one single diagnostic test was available to perform in this patient what would it be, and how should it be interpreted?
iii. In this patient, basal T3 and T4 were unusually elevated. What is the most likely explanation?

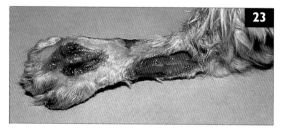

23 A young, adult male, outdoor cat was presented for a second opinion. The owners reported the cat had had a nonhealing wound on the hind leg for over 2 months (23). Previous skin biopsy findings were consistent with a bacterial pyoderma; however, lesions did not respond to appropriate antibiotic therapy. Impression smears of the lesion and cultures did not grow any fungal or atypical mycobacterial organisms. The lesion started with a bite wound, and over the last several months had progressed. On physical examination, periodontal disease and stomatitis were present; however, the owners were not aware if this was a recent event. The only other findings on physical examination were marked weight loss, mild dehydration, and an oily matted hair coat. Before performing any further dermatological testing, what screening tests are indicated in this cat?

22 i. Canine hypothyroidism. The most common causes of naturally acquired hypo-thyroidism in dogs are lymphocytic thyroiditis (which is genetically programmed) and idiopathic thyroid necrosis and atrophy. Diagnosis of hypothyroidism can be difficult and expensive, particularly if the patient is exhibiting nondermatological signs. In these patients, complete blood counts, serum chemistry panels, urinalyses, and skin biopsies may be needed to narrow the differential diagnoses. In this patient, the clinical suspicion is high; therefore, thyroid function testing would be an appropriate first diagnostic.

ii. The single most reliable test for hypothyroidism is a thyroid biopsy (which is impractical excluding situations where a tumor is expected). Although tempting in this patient, response to thyroid hormone supplementation as a diagnostic test is not recommended. Evaluation of thyroid hormone supplementation is unreliable since thyroid hormone supplementation will produce changes in attitude, activity obesity, and hair growth in nonhypothyroid dogs. Furthermore, the administration of a thyroid hormone supplement to euthyroid dogs is not without risk; complications from iatrogenic hyperthyroidism can occur.

Thyroid function testing using TSH is cost effective and routinely performed. Unfortunately, bovine TSH is not available worldwide, and human TSH is too expensive to be used routinely. Thus, thyrotropin releasing hormone is an alternative function test. Normal dogs show a 1.2-fold increase in T4 above the baseline, assuming the baseline samples are within normal range. Because so many factors can affect thyroid hormone concentrations, simultaneous measurement of multiple thyroid hormone concentrations is recommended. Measurement of fT4 concentrations by dialysis is the most accurate single test, but this test is expensive and not always available. In general, single measurements of T3 or T4 are rarely diagnostic unless they are within the upper limits of normal. The author recommends evaluating a combination of fT4, T4, and cTSH concentrations, along with consideration of the dog's clinical signs. This dog was hypothyroid.

iii. If basal T4 and T3 concentrations were unexpectedly elevated, the most likely explanation would be the presence of T3 and/or T4 antibodies.

23 This is a male outdoor cat with a history of a nonhealing wound. In addition, the cat is showing early signs of systemic illness (i.e. weight loss, dehydration, matted hair coat). It should be tested for FeLV and/or FIV. This cat was FeLV-positive and was also severely anemic upon further testing. Skin diseases associated with both of these two immunosuppressive feline viruses include recurrent bacterial skin infections, nonhealing wounds, exfoliative dermatitis, generalized pruritus, recurrent abscesses, chronic dermatophytosis, demodicosis, and oral disease.

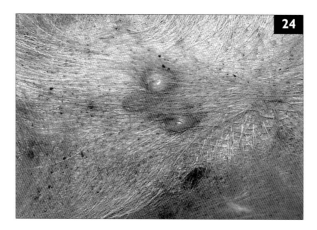

24 An intact pustule on the ventral abdomen of a dog with a superficial bacterial pyoderma is shown (24).

i. If a bacterial culture of this lesion was performed, what primary pathogen would be expected to be found? What is the difference between 'resident' and 'transient' flora?

ii. What enzymes and toxins are produced by pathogenic staphylococci?

iii. What is the relationship between enzymes, toxins, and virulence factors in the development of bacterial pyoderma?

25 A dog was presented for a 'rash' on the ventral abdomen (25). Physical examination revealed lesions on the ventrum, medial thigh, and lateral thorax region. Close examination of the patient revealed intact papules, pustules, crusted pustules, and epidermal collarettes. Skin scraping and flea combings were negative.

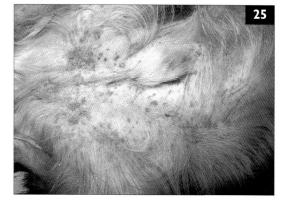

i. What is the clinical diagnosis?

ii. This infection will require 21–30 days of antibiotic therapy; infections are treated for at least 1 week past clinical cure. What makes an 'ideal' antibiotic for treatment of bacterial pyoderma?

iii. List the antibiotics that are suitable for 'first occurrence or empirical therapy', and list the antibiotics that are suitable for recurrent or deep pyodermas.

24, 25: Answers

24 i. *Staphylococcus intermedius*. This is a Gram-positive, beta hemolytic, coagulase-positive cocci. This organism is probably the primary cutaneous pathogen of cats too. Bacteria cultured from normal skin are considered to be normal inhabitants of the skin. They may be resident flora (organisms that successfully multiply on healthy skin) or transients (organisms that do not usually multiply on normal skin). There is debate as to whether or not *S. intermedius* is part of the resident or transient flora. Regardless, overgrowth of normal bacterial flora that results in clinical disease requires medical treatment.

ii. Toxins and enzymes produced by pathogenic staphylococci include toxin TSS-1 (toxic shock syndrome-1), which causes toxic syndrome in people; protein A, which is able to bind the Fc portion of immunoglobulins with pro-inflammatory effects; the enzyme coagulase, which allows for the deposition of fibrin on bacterial cells inhibiting the ability of neutrophils and macrophages; and beta-lactamase, which is responsive for resistance against nonprotected penicillins (Noli, 2002).

iii. To date, no difference has been found between the toxins and enzymes from bacterial isolates from healthy dogs and dogs with bacterial pyoderma. However, a difference in the production of a virulence factor that facilitates the adherence of bacteria to host skin has been noted. Pathogenic bacteria show increased adhesion to extracellular matrix proteins when compared to bacteria from normal dogs (McEwan, 2000; Noli, 2002).

25 i. Superficial bacterial pyoderma. The clinical signs are classic for bacterial pyoderma. In this patient all of the clinical stages of a pyoderma are present: papule, pustule, crusted papule/pustule, and epidermal collarette. The most common clinical signs of deep pyoderma are blood, pus, matting of the hair coat, and cutaneous pain. These are absent, as are hemorrhagic bullae; therefore, a deep bacterial infection is not present.

ii. Antibiotics should have a spectrum of activity that includes *Staphylococcus intermedius*, reach high skin concentrations, be bactericidal, have few adverse effects, should be easy to administer, unlikely to cause bacterial resistance, and be inexpensive (Noli, 2002).

iii. First occurrence superficial bacterial pyoderma cases can almost always be treated empirically. The two most common reasons to do a bacterial culture and sensitivity in these patients are the finding of a mixed bacterial population on cytological examination, or knowledge that the animal has a previous history of antibiotic therapy for other reasons. Erythromycin, lincomycin, clindamycin, and trimethoprim-sulfa are common first choice antibiotics for empirical therapy. Cephalosporin, amoxicillin with clavulanic acid, and fluoroquinolone antibiotics are used in cases of deep pyoderma. Treatment should be based upon culture and sensitivity in these cases.

26 A 9-month-old cat was presented for a routine health examination after being adopted from an animal shelter. The unique coloring of the cat's hair coat especially impressed the owners, particularly the 'white tips' on the ends of the hairs (26a). The owners reported the cat to be mildly pruritic. Flea combings were done, and an organism was found; several of the hairs with white tips were examined microscopically. The only other pet in the house was a dog, which was unaffected.

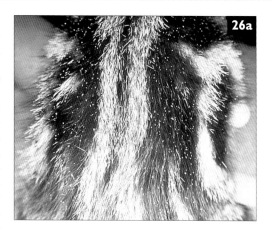

i. A microscopic view of a 'white tip' on the cat's coat is shown (26b), and of an organism (26c) found on flea combing of the hair coat. What are these organisms, and how should the cat be treated?

ii. Three days after treating the cat, the owner calls. Both of her children have been diagnosed with 'what the cat has'! The owner is very agitated that she was not warned of the zoonotic implications. What are the zoonotic implications of this cat's infestation?

iii. What is the genus and species of this organism, and what is unique about it in cats? Why is this parasite more common in the winter than in the summer?

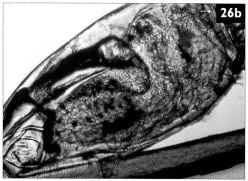

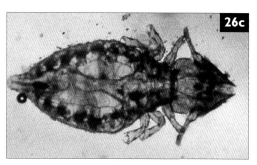

27 What are the three major categories of animal shampoos?

26, 27: Answers

26 i. Louse and louse egg or 'nit' cemented to the hair shaft. This cat has pediculosis. The cat should be washed to remove mechanically as many of the lice and louse nits as possible prior to treatment. Removal of the louse nits can be facilitated with a rinse of a 1:4 dilution of household white vinegar in water; this loosens the cement attachment of the nit to the hair. A thorough washing with a flea shampoo should follow. After the cat is dry, it should be treated for 30 days with a flea control product labeled for use in cats. Topical spot-on products as sole therapy are best avoided; a thorough spraying of the hair coat is needed. The author has found fipronil spray repeated again in 30 days is very effective. Ivermectin is effective if used at a dose of 200 µg/kg orally or subcutaneously every 2 weeks for 6 weeks. Imidacloprid spot-on is effective, but it is important to repeat treatments and to remove mechanically lice and louse eggs from the hairs to ensure eradication.

ii. Lice are host specific, and the children were not infested from the cat. Lice can act as an intermediate host for *Dipylidium caninum*, the dog tapeworm. Although rare, people can become infected with *D. caninum*; this most commonly occurs in children that play with infected dogs or cats (Turner, 1962). Infected people may develop abdominal pain, anorexia, diarrhea, and anal pruritus.

iii. Cats have only one species of louse that infests them, the biting louse, *Felicola subrostratuas*. The reproductive system of the louse is affected by temperature. In the winter, the temperature in the hair coat and on the skin surface is most conducive to louse fecundity. In the summer, the temperature at the surface of the skin can be significantly higher than the ambient temperature; the higher temperature at the skin surface has an inhibitory effect on reproduction of lice.

27 Cleansing, antiparasiticidal, and 'medicated' shampoos. The purpose of cleansing shampoos is to remove dirt and debris from the hair coat. These are commonly sold over the counter as 'grooming shampoos'. Antiparasiticidal shampoos are essentially 'flea shampoos'. They are essentially a cleansing shampoo with an added anti-parasiticidal drug (e.g. pyrethrins). The amount of insecticide in the shampoo is too small to be effective as a primary method of parasite control. 'Medicated' shampoos can be subdivided into several groups depending upon the primary activity or active ingredient. Antimicrobial shampoos are used to treat bacterial or fungal (usually *Malassezia*) infections. Common antibacterial agents are chlorhexidine and benzoyl peroxide. Common antifungal shampoos may contain chlorhexidine, ketoconazole, or miconazole. Antipruritic shampoos are usually a combination of a cleansing shampoo and an anti-inflammatory agent such as 1% hydrocortisone, 2% diphenhydramine, 1% pramoxine, or colloidal oatmeal. Antiseborrheic shampoos contain salicylic acid, sulfur, tar, or selenium sulfide.

28 A 10-year-old male mixed breed dog is presented for evaluation of a mass in the right axilla. The owners report that the mass has been slow to develop and has been bothersome to the dog only recently. The location and size of the mass are making it difficult for the dog to walk. Physical examination reveals a firm 10 cm diameter mass in the right caudal axilla. The skin over the mass is freely moveable; however, the mass is firmly attached to

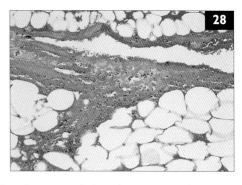

the tissue beneath. A FNA is performed and it is noted that the specimen disappears after being dipped into the fixative. A tissue biopsy of the mass is obtained prior to surgical removal. A photomicrograph of a section of the skin biopsy is shown (28).

i. Based upon the history, FNA findings, and skin biopsy, what is the diagnosis, and what is the treatment of choice? A tentative diagnosis can often be made in-house. How is that done?

ii. What is an infiltrative lipoma, and how does it differ from a 'lipoma'?

iii. Is calcium chloride a treatment option in this case?

29 The head and neck of a middle-aged cocker spaniel dog with a history of seborrhea are shown (29). The dog was presented for evaluation of multi-focal areas of hair loss and pigmentation. The hyperpigmentation is, in fact, an area of thick crusting that can be peeled off to reveal an erythematous moist area. Careful examination revealed numerous other lesions like this on the dorsum. Pustules, papules, and epidermal collarettes are present on the ventrum. This lesion is com-

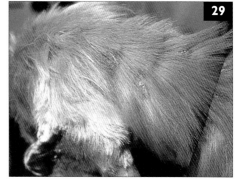

mon in cocker spaniel dogs, especially those with primary seborrhea.

i. What is the clinical diagnosis? What diagnostic tests are indicated? The owner has financial constraints and refuses diagnostic tests; what therapy should be recommended based upon the clinical diagnosis?

ii. What would the histological description of a biopsy specimen from a dog with primary seborrhea be expected to report?

iii. What adverse effects can occur with the use of tar-based shampoos?

28 i. Lipoma. This is the most common skin tumor of dogs with surgical removal being the treatment of choice. Lipomas do not need to be surgically removed unless the mass is causing a mechanical problem for the dog. Lipomas in the caudal axillary area are common in dogs and can cause difficulties with locomotion. FNA of a lipoma will often reveal an acellular aspirate that glistens. When the specimen is placed into routine fixative, the lipid dissolves.

ii. An infiltrative lipoma is an uncommon neoplasm with a predilection for the limbs. These tumors, unlike the typical lipoma, are large, poorly circumscribed, soft, deep masses that invade between muscles, fascial planes, tendons, and even into joint capsules. These tumors are associated with dysfunction and pain. They are most common in the Labrador retriever and doberman pinscher breeds. Complete surgical excision is difficult.

iii. Intralesional injection of 10% calcium chloride will cause regression of the lesion, but it is not recommended as a treatment because it causes irritation and necrosis.

29 i. Superficial bacterial pyoderma causing a 'seborrheic plaque'. Diagnostic tests should include skin scrapings for mites, impression smears to look for concurrent yeast infections and, possibly, a dermatophyte culture. Treating skin diseases without adequate confirmation of the diagnosis is always a less than satisfactory approach to patient care. Canine pyoderma frequently is a clinical diagnosis; impression smears are needed to see if there are concurrent yeast infections.

The most likely diagnosis in this dog is a bacterial infection with a possible secondary yeast infection. These hyperpigmented seborrheic plaques are very common in dogs with primary seborrhea and are caused by bacterial infections. Careful examination of the patient may reveal scales piercing hairs, another common clinical sign of a bacterial infection. One cost effective strategy would be to treat the dog with oral cephalexin for 30 days and have the owner bathe the dog daily in ketoconazole or a combination antibacterial/antifungal shampoo to treat for the presumed secondary yeast infection. If there is inadequate response to therapy in 30 days, diagnostic testing will be needed.

ii. In an uncomplicated case of primary seborrhea, the most common histological findings would include: hyperplastic, superficial, perivascular dermatitis with ortho- or parakeratotic hyperkeratosis. The thickness of the basal cell layer is usually disproportionate to the thickness of the cornified epitheilium; the basal cell layer is only 1–3 cells thick while there is marked hyperkeratosis present. None of these key clinical signs may be seen if the skin site surface is wiped, scrubbed, or tampered with prior to biopsy.

iii. Tar is odorous, potentially irritating, photosensitizing, and carcinogenic (Scott *et al.*, 2001d).

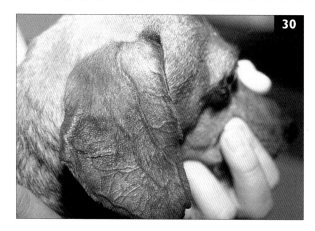

30 A 5-year-old dachshund dog with bilateral pinnal alopecia is shown (30). The hair loss has been slowly progressive, is limited to the ear pinnae, and the dog is nonpruritic. Skin scrapings are negative, as are fungal cultures. A skin biopsy revealed dimunitive hair follicles.
i. What is the most likely cause?
ii. There are four classic syndromes in dogs with this disorder. What are they?

31 A photomicrograph of normal dog skin is shown (31).
i. What are the three major layers of the skin and the layers of the epidermis?
ii. What adnexal structures are produced in the skin?
iii. What are tylotrich hairs, and where are they located?

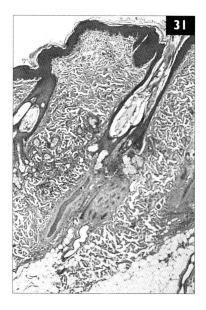

30 i. The most likely cause is canine pinnal alopecia or pattern baldness. This is a commonly observed condition in such breeds as dachshunds, chihuahuas, Boston terriers, whippets, and Italian greyhounds. It can also be seen in cats. The cause is unknown, but it is most likely a heritable condition. No treatment is needed, as this is considered a cosmetic disorder. There are anecdotal reports that the condition may respond to oral melatonin (3–6 mg q8h).

ii. The first syndrome is shown in this case, pinnal alopecia. The second syndrome occurs in American and Portuguese water spaniel dogs and is characterized by hair loss on the ventral neck, caudomedial thighs, and tail beginning about 6 months of age. The third syndrome occurs in greyhound dogs, and affected dogs lose their hair on the lateral thighs. This must be differentiated from bald thigh syndrome in greyhounds, which usually has an endocrine cause. The final syndrome is seen in breeds such as dachshunds, Boston terriers, chihuahuas, whippets, Manchester terriers, and greyhounds. At about 6 months of age, affected dogs lose their hair on the post-auricular area, ventral neck, and ventrum (Scott *et al.*, 2001h).

31 i. The three major layers of the skin are the epidermis, dermis, and hypodermis (subcutis or panniculus). The layers of the epidermis from proximal to distal are the stratum basale, stratum spinosum, stratum granulosum, stratum lucidum, and stratum corneum. The stratum basale, or basal layer rests upon the basement membrane and is responsible for the production of new epidermal cells. In the spinous or prickle cell layer, the keratinocyte cytoskeleton is produced. In the stratum granulosum or granular layer, keratohyalin is produced and deposited. Cells in this layer are flattened and basophilic, and 'granules' can be seen in the cytoplasm. Cells in the stratum lucidum or 'clear layer', are anuclear, and this layer is rich in protein-bound lipids. This layer is best developed in footpads and can also be seen in the nasal planum. It is not seen in other areas of the skin. The most distal layer or stratum corneum, is the skin layer in contact with the environment. It is the fully cornified layer and is made of flattened, anuclear, densely packed keratinocytes.

ii. The skin produces hairs and hair follicles, sebaceous glands, sweat glands, specialized glands (i.e. anal sacs, tail gland, glands of the external ear canal, and circumanal glands), claws, nails, and the horny layer of the skin.

iii. Tylotrich hairs are large hair follicles scattered throughout the body. The hairs are larger than normal hairs and contain one large hair surrounded by a complex of neurovascular tissue at the level of the sebaceous gland. They are believed to be rapid adapting mechanoreceptors.

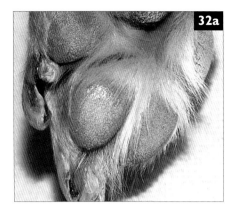
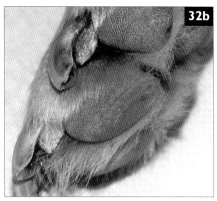

32 A 5-year-old mixed breed dog was presented for lameness and sloughing (onychomadesis) of all of the nails. The owner reported that the lesions started on one paw, and then gradually developed on all four paws over 2–3 months. Examination revealed the nails were separating at the claw bed exposing the vascular corium (quick) (32a, b). Nails that had sloughed and regrown were misshapen, soft (onychomalacia), and brittle. The footpads were normal and there were no other signs of skin disease. Previous fungal cultures were negative, and the condition did not respond to a 4 week course of oral antibiotics. The third digit of an affected dewclaw was amputated and submitted for histological examination. The biopsy report found lichenoid interface dermatitis.

i. What is the most likely diagnosis?

ii. How should this be treated?

iii. List the most common parasitic, infectious, immune-mediated, and neoplastic diseases that affect the claw.

33 The owner of the dog shown complained the dog's ear tips 'do not heal'. According to the owner, there is no history of trauma to the ear tip. However, the ear tips intermittently ulcerate, bleed, crust, and then heal very slowly. The ear margin is cracked, fissured, and slightly deformed although much of the lesion is hidden because of the hair coat (33). The dog has no other history of skin disease.

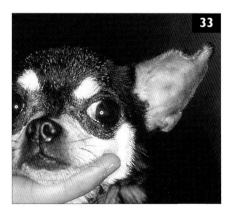

i. What is this lesion?

ii. What is the most common etiology?

iii. How should this lesion be managed?

32 i. Lichenoid interface dermatitis is most often associated with immune-mediated diseases, particularly lupus. Lupoid dermatoses can be localized to the face (e.g. 'classic' cutaneous lupus-erythematosus), the face and skin, a region of the body (nails), or generalized (i.e. systemic lupus erythematosus). In this case, the most likely diagnosis is symmetric lupoid onychodystrophy. The biopsy findings are compatible with lupoid dermatitis, and the lesions involve all four feet, hence the name 'symmetric lupoid onychodystrophy'. Currently, it is unknown if this is a specific disease entity or a reaction pattern. The latter is most likely, and there may be numerous triggers. Overvaccination has been proposed as a possible cause, but no evidence to confirm this has been published. Anecdotal reports indicate some of these cases may be triggered by food allergies.

ii. These dogs are very lame, and they often snag avulsed nails on carpeting or while walking. The sloughing nail should be avulsed and removed under general anesthesia, if necessary. Mild cases can be treated with a combination of tetracycline and niacinamide, or essential fatty acids (omega-3 and omega-6 fatty acids). Severely affected dogs respond to oral glucocorticoids within a few weeks. The author uses a combination of glucocorticoids and pentoxifylline for 4–6 weeks until the sloughing halts, and then continues with pentoxifylline therapy alone. Although more expensive, cyclosporin A is another option for therapy and may be as effective as prednisone. Systemic anti-inflammatory therapy varies depending upon the severity of the lesions; if therapy is stopped symptoms will recur, and if the underlying cause remains unknown.

iii. Parasitic causes include demodicosis, hookworm dermatitis, and leishmaniasis. Infectious causes include bacterial and yeast infections along with dermatophytes, such as *Trichophyton* spp. infections. The intermediate and deep mycoses (blastomycosis, cryptococcosis, and sporotrichosis) can also cause disease. Lupus erythematosus, bullous pemphigoid, and pemphigus vulgaris can cause claw disorders while pemphigus foliaceus usually causes purulent paronychia and footpad hyperkeratosis. Neoplastic diseases associated with the claw include squamous cell carcinoma, subungual keratoacanthoma, inverted papillomas, and sweat gland carcinomas.

33 i. Ear tip necrosis.
ii. Vasculitis or thromboembolism.
iii. These cases are difficult to manage as cycles of active necrosis and healing occur repeatedly. Laser surgery can repair the cosmetic defect, but there is a high risk of lesions developing yet again. In cases of thromboembolism, surgery may be helpful. Dogs with vasculitis may respond to glucocorticoids and/or pentoxifylline.

34 The owners of a pet store presented this puppy for examination for primarily 'behavioral reasons'. The puppy was irritable, growling, restless, and 'jittery'. Upon careful questioning, the owners reported that the puppy scratched more than others in the litter. Physical examination of the puppy was normal except for the skin, which was scaly, odorous, and clearly pruritic. Macroscopic white organisms were found when the puppy's thick coat was

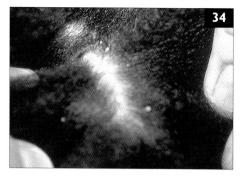

parted (34). The organisms were slow moving and many were attached to the skin.
i. What is the most likely diagnosis, and how can the diagnosis be confirmed?
ii. This parasite is divided into two major groups. What are they, how does this division affect the clinical presentation of the disease, and what is the most likely species infesting this puppy?
iii. What other parasites can appear as white and macroscopic?

35 An adult Himalayan cat was presented for an emergency examination because the cat was vomiting and not eating. The cat has a history of eating string, and the owner was concerned the cat had ingested another linear foreign body. On physical examination, no string was found in the mouth. During the examination, the cat vomited a malodorous liquid that smelled like feces. Palpation of the cat's abdomen revealed a large amount of feces in the large bowel. The owner reported that the cat had had increas-

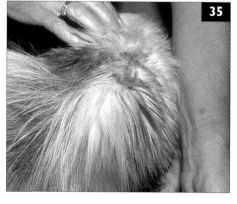

ing problems with 'hair balls' over the last month. When questioned further, the owner reported the cat has been shedding more than normal and was pruritic. Diffuse hyperpigmentation on the skin was noted along with a sparse hair coat (35). As the cat was being put back into its carrier, a raised erythematous lesion was noted on the owner's arm.
i. What is the most likely cause of this cat's constipation and vomiting? What are the most likely differential diagnoses for the skin disease presented?
ii. What diagnostic tests should be recommended?
iii. What should the owner be told about her skin lesions?

34 i. Pediculosis or louse infestation. Lice are most common in animals that are overcrowded and/or debilitated. This is often a disease of neglect. Infested animals often have a dirty matted hair coat and a 'mousey' odor. Diagnosis can be made via visual examination because lice are large parasitic insects. Lice can be captured with flea combs or via acetate tape preparations and examined with magnification.

ii. Lice are divided into two suborders: Anoplura (sucking lice) and Mallophaga (biting lice). Biting lice move rapidly on the host, often scurrying into the hair coat when parted for examination, while sucking lice move more slowly and are easier to capture. Biting lice cause more irritation because they move around more on the host and feed on epidermal debris. Animals may be irritable and, if infested with a sucking louse, anemic. Pruritus may range from mild to severe. Dogs are commonly infested with one of two species of lice: *Linognathus setosus* (sucking louse) or *Trichodectes canis* (biting louse). The latter may act as an intermediate host for the dog tapeworm, *Dipylidium caninum*. Because these lice were slow moving and attached to the skin, they were most likely sucking lice or *L. setosus*.

iii. Other parasites that can appear as 'white' are *Dermanyssus gallinae* (poultry mite), *Cheyletiella* spp., and *Lynxacarus radovsky*.

35 i. Hair impaction in the large colon. Pruritic cats and/or cats with skin diseases that make the hairs fragile often have current problems with constipation and/or hair balls, due to increased ingestion of hair. This cat's primary dermatological problem is pruritus; therefore, the most likely differential diagnoses include: dermatophytosis, fleas or flea allergy dermatitis, cheyletiellosis, demodicosis, atopy, and food allergy. Yeast and bacterial pyoderma are possible causes of pruritus, but they are most likely to be secondary to another underlying disease. Bacterial pyoderma in cats is considered a 'rare' disease if one looks for the classic clinical signs expected in dogs: intact pustules, epidermal collarettes, and multifocal areas of hair loss. In the author's experience, the most common symptoms of bacterial pyoderma in cats include scaling, especially over the lumbosacral area, scales pierced by hairs, retained matted hair coat, miliary dermatitis, and follicular plugging. Many of these cats have concurrent bacterial and yeast infections and respond to oral antibiotics and itraconazole.

ii. Skin scrapings to rule out demodicosis, flea combings to look for fleas, lice, and *Cheyletiella* mites, impression smears to look for yeast and/or bacteria, and a dermatophyte culture. This cat had dermatophytosis due to *Microsporum canis*. Hyperpigmentation of the skin is rare in cats and is seen most commonly in dermatophytosis. A large tricobezoar was removed surgically, and the hairs were culture-positive for *M. canis*.

iii. The owner should be informed that this is a zoonotic skin disease and referred to her physician.

36 The owner of a 3-year-old male cat with a lesion presented the cat for a first opinion. The owner reports the lesion had been present for over 1 year and tends to come and go, always recurring in the same area. The lesion is localized to the cat's left lateral foreleg (36). The owner has not developed any skin lesions after handling the cat, and the other two cats in the house are normal.

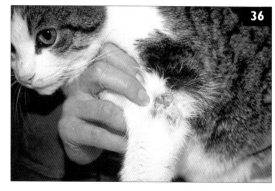

i. What is the cat's dermatological problem, and what are the differential diagnoses?
ii. What diagnostic tests are indicated?
iii. List the most commonly used drugs for the treatment of anxiety or compulsive behavior in small animal dermatology, their drug class, and their mode of action.

37 A middle-aged dog is presented for the complaint of 'hard skin'. The owners reports the dog had developed 'rock hard skin lumps' over the last 6 months. Most of the lesions do not seem to bother the dog; however, a few are very exudative and pruritic, and the dog chews at these lesions. Physical examination reveals a depressed, panting, pot-bellied dog with a history of polyuria, polydipsia, and polyphagia. On

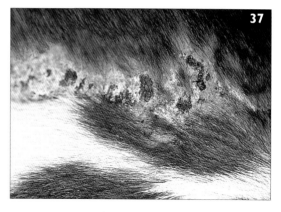

dermatological examination, there are numerous erythematous areas of hair loss and a white particulate material in these areas. Palpation of these areas reveals well-demarcated raised hard plaques (37). These raised plaques are generalized but seem to be most numerous on the dorsum and in the axillary and inguinal regions. The dog traumatizes all of the sites it can reach, suggesting that the dog is pruritic. The hair coat is thinning.
i. What is the most likely diagnosis for the skin lesions?
ii. How can the dogs' pruritus be accounted for?
iii. What other diseases could cause these lesions in the skin?

36, 37: Answers

36 i. The dermatological problem is a nonhealing wound. The differential diagnoses include self-trauma due to the irritation or discomfort from parasitic infestations (fleas, *Cheyletiella*, lice, *Demodex*), bacterial infections, superficial or intermediate fungal infections, and allergic skin diseases. Because the lesion is unilateral and recurs in the same location, self-trauma in response to pain (soft tissue or bone), a foreign body, or neoplasia (e.g. mast cell tumor) must be considered along with psychogenic self-trauma.
ii. Diagnostic tests include skin scrapings, flea combings, trial of flea control, impression smears, dermatophyte culture, radiographs, and a skin biopsy. All of these tests were normal or negative. The owner declined evaluation for allergies; however, the lesion did not respond to glucocorticoids suggesting that pruritus, as would be seen in an allergic disease, was not the underlying cause of the discomfort. This was eventually diagnosed as a case of self-trauma or psychogenic dermatitis. The cat's lesion resolved with clomipramine, but recurred when the medication was discontinued. The self-mutilation stopped when the owner's roommate moved out.
iii. Commonly used tricyclic antidepressants are amitriptyline, clomipramine, and doxepin. Citalopram, fluvoxamine, fluoxetine, and paroxetine are specific serotonin reuptake inhibitors. All of these drugs work by selectively inhibiting the uptake of serotonin. Hydrocordone is a narcotic and optiate agonist (Juarbe-Diaz and Frank, 2002).

37 i. Calcinosis cutis. This patient had hyperadrenocorticism.
ii. Lesions of calcinosis cutis can be very inflammatory and may cause pain and pruritus. It is usually assumed that dogs with calcinosis cutis secondary to hyperadrenocorticism will not be pruritic; however, this is not always the case. Often the sites resemble areas of deep pyoderma and are pruritic to the patient. There is no specific treatment for calcinosis cutis. Lesions resolve when the underlying cause is addressed and treated (iatrogenic or spontaneously occurring hyperadrenocorticism). Resolving lesions of calcinosis cutis can become very pruritic and often require secondary antimicrobial treatment. Intensely pruritic dogs may benefit from cyclosporin A therapy or short-term application of a low-dose dexamethasone spray to relieve the discomfort. Depending upon the cause of the calcinosis cutis, it may take weeks to months to resolve.
iii. Calcinosis cutis can be either dystrophic calcification or metastatic calcification. The most common cause of the latter is chronic renal disease. Dystrophic causes include calcinosis circumscripta, inflammation, or infection (e.g. calcification of the ear canal of dogs), degenerative lesions, or neoplasia. Calcinosis cutis can be seen in dogs with diabetes mellitus, and in puppies with acute severe infection or inflammation.

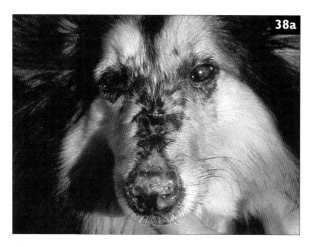

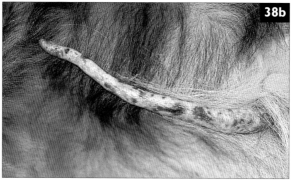

38 A 3-year-old, intact, female Shetland sheepdog is presented for the problem of hair loss on the face (38a) and tail tip (38b). The facial lesions and alopecia of the tail are not pruritic. These lesions first developed when she was 16 weeks of age and have gradually progressed. Skin scrapings have been consistently negative for *Demodex* mites, and repeated fungal cultures were negative. Several other littermates had similar lesions and a contagion was suspected but none found. Finally, the lesions did not respond to oral antibiotic therapy. The owners report that she is a 'sloppy eater' and has never had regular heat cycles.

i. Based upon the information provided, what is the most likely diagnosis and what other clinical signs are commonly associated with this disease?

ii. How is this disease diagnosed?

iii. This is a heritable disease. What is the mode of transmission, and how is this disease treated?

38: Answer

38 i. Familial canine dermatomyositis of Shetland sheepdogs and collie dogs. Clinical signs can occur as early as 7 weeks of age in these dogs, and may consist of hair loss and erythema around the eyes, on the ear tips, metatarsal and metacarpal areas, digits, and on the tip of the tail. Myositis is a feature of this disease and varies from mild to severe. Dogs with more severe signs may present with a history of difficulty in chewing and/or swallowing (sloppy eater), a high 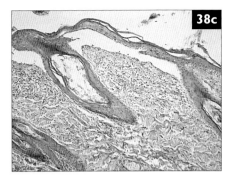 stepping gait, megaesophagus, and/or aspiration pneumonia. The most common signs of myositis are atrophy of the muscles of mastication and hind limbs.

ii. A clinical diagnosis can be made based upon the history, breed, clinical signs, and ruling out other common causes of follicular dermatitis in young dogs. In this disease, typical lesions usually develop before 6 months of age. Differential diagnoses include: dermatophytosis, bacterial pyoderma, and demodicosis. These are easily ruled out via skin scrapings, dermatophyte culture, and response to treatment. Other differential diagnoses include cutaneous lupus erythematosus and EBS. Lupus erythematosus usually occurs in older dogs. EBS is a rare disease, and affected animals have bullous lesions on the skin and in the oral mucosa. In canine dermatomyositis, supportive findings for the diagnosis can be found on skin biopsy, muscle biopsy, and muscle conduction studies, or EMG. Skin biopsy findings show hydropic degeneration of basal cells, intrabasalar or subepidermal clefting, pigmentary incontinence, follicular atrophy, and possibly vasculitis (38c). Muscle biopsy findings show inflammatory exudates, muscle fiber necrosis, and muscle atrophy. Needle EMG abnormalities include positive sharp waves and fibrillation potentials in muscles of the head and distal extremities. Definitive skin and muscle biopsy specimens are often difficult to obtain.

iii. This is a hereditary disease, and affected animals should not be bred. Breeding studies have shown an autosomal dominant mode of inheritance. The goal of treatment is to minimize the worsening of clinical signs and maintain a good quality of life for the dogs. Mild clinical signs can be managed with oral vitamin E (200–800 IU/day), which may help the skin lesions but not the muscle lesions. Animals with moderate disease and/or relapsing episodes from sun exposure or trauma may benefit from prednisone (1–2 mg/kg PO), and severely affected dogs may require chronic prednisone therapy. Pentoxifylline (200–400 mg PO q24h–q48h) has been helpful in some dogs to minimize or eliminate the need for glucocorticoid therapy.

39 A 12-week-old puppy was presented for examination because of 'pimples' under its forelimbs (39).

i. What is this lesion, and what is the common name for this skin disease in puppies?

ii. What would a cytological smear of an intact pustule be expected to show, and what is the controversy regarding treatment of 'puppy impetigo'?

iii. 'Impetigo' is most commonly seen in puppies. Describe the clinical characteristics of this disease's counterpart in kittens and in adult dogs.

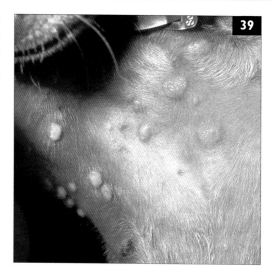

40 An obese 6-year-old male collie dog is presented for pain and sloughing skin that developed over the last 3 weeks. Note the ulcerations and erosions (40). The lesions began as flaccid bullae that ruptured and coalesced to form the lesions seen. The owner reports a similar, but milder, episode occurred last summer that spontaneously resolved. Close examination of the patient reveals small ulcerative lesions are present on the eyelids, inner pinnae, anus, and footpads. The lesions are painful upon palpation. Skin biopsy findings reveal hydropic degeneration of basal cells, vesicles at the dermoepidermal junction, and lichenoid dermatitis. Hair follicles are normal. DIF and ANA testing are negative.

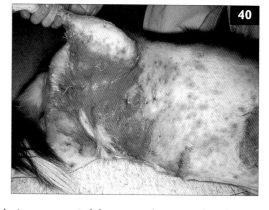

i. What skin diseases unique to collie dogs and Shetland sheepdogs could present like this?

ii. Of these diseases, which is most likely?

iii. How is this disease managed?

39 i. This is a pustule. This condition is also called 'puppy pyoderma' or puppy impetigo'. Impetigo is characterized by large, rapidly developing, subcorneal pustules affecting sparsely haired areas of the skin, especially in the flexor areas.

ii. Impetigo in puppies occurs in the axillary and inguinal regions. It is diagnosed via clinical presentation and/or impression smears. Impression smears of intact pustules reveal neutrophils and keratinocytes may be seen. Depending upon the sample site, cocci may be visible intra- or extracellularly. The controversy regarding treatment of this syndrome revolves around the administration of systemic antibiotics since clinical signs may resolve without antibiotic treatment in some puppies. Impetigo in other puppies may resolve with only topical therapy (e.g. daily antibacterial baths with chlorhexidine) while others may require up to 21 days of oral antibiotics. Benzoyl peroxide is best avoided in pediatric patients as it can be very irritating.

iii. Impetigo is rare in kittens, but it can be seen on the neck of kittens that are 'mouthed' excessively by the queen. The pustular lesions are very transient in kittens, and owners usually present young kittens for the complaint of crusting and matting of the hair on the neck. It is uncommon to see clusters of intact pustules on adult dogs. However, the discovery of large numbers of intact pustules should raise the suspicion of a possible autoimmune skin disease characterized by pustules (e.g. pemphigus). Bullous impetigo in adult dogs has been seen in association with hyperadrenocorticism, diabetes mellitus, hypothyroidism, and other systemic illnesses (Scott *et al.*, 2001b).

40 i. The breed-related skin diseases include SLE, dermatomyositis, BP, and idiopathic ulcerative dermatitis.

ii. Idiopathic ulcerative dermatitis of Shetland sheepdogs and collie dogs. Clinically, these lesions are compatible with BP or SLE. However, DIF and ANA testing were negative, and the skin biopsy findings were incompatible. In addition, SLE and BP diseases usually do not wax and wane or spontaneously resolve. The clinical lesions are incompatible with dermatomyositis because this disease is not ulcerative. A common biopsy finding in dermatomytosis is follicular atrophy, not lichenoid dermatitis or clefting. Finally, dogs with this disease tend to show lesions at a young age and/or have a history of previous skin disease.

iii. Idiopathic ulcerative dermatitis of Shetland sheepdogs and collie dogs tends to have a cyclic nature; the disease is often worse in summer suggesting that sun exposure is a trigger. Trauma can worsen lesions, and every effort to minimize trauma should be made. Antibiotic therapy is needed if a secondary bacterial infection is present. Glucocorticoids, pentoxifylline, azathioprine, Vitamin E, and tetracycline and niacinamide have been anecdotally reported to be effective. This disease may be a variant of lupus erythematosus and 'vesicular cutaneous lupus erythematosus' has been proposed as a new name.

41 A photomicrograph of positive direct immunofluorescence testing from a skin biopsy in a dog is shown (**41**).
i. What pattern of immunofluorescence is shown?
ii. What autoimmune skin diseases show this pattern?

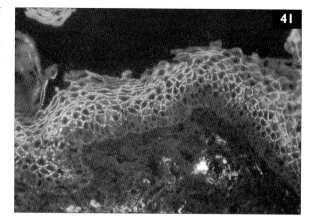

42 What is the difference between eumycotic mycetoma, actinomycotic mycetoma, and pseudomycetoma?

43 The dorsal back of a 5-year-old male intact schnauzer dog is shown (**43**). The dog has just been diagnosed with atopy. The owner reports that the dog has had 'bumps' over its dorsum almost its entire life. Palpation of the dorsum reveals diffuse, sharp, crusted papules from the neck to the lumbosacral area. When the hair coat is clipped, numerous comedones are seen.
i. What is the common name for the lesions on the dog's back?
ii. How does it relate to the dog's atopy?
iii. How is it treated?

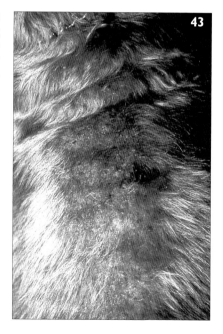

41 i. The pattern is intercellular immunofluorescence.

ii. This pattern of immunofluorescence is most commonly associated with the pemphigus complex (PF, pemphigus erythematosus, pemphigus vulgaris). Pemphigus erythematosus may show both intercellular and basement membrane deposition of antibodies.

42 The terminology regarding 'mycetomas' is very confusing. A mycetoma is subcutaneous infection that usually presents as a nodular lesion. Classic lesions are raised, nodular, cool to the touch, and have open draining tracks exuding 'tissue granules or grains'. The latter are formed as a result of host antibody reaction. Eumycotic mycetomas are caused by by either pigmented (dematiaceous) or nonpigmented fungi. Actinomycotic mycetomas are caused by bacteria of the Actinomycetales order such as *Actinomyces* or *Nocardia*. Pseudomycetomas, another confusing term, are caused by dermatophytes or bacterial infections such as *Staphylococcus* spp.

43 i. The common name for this condition is 'schnauzer comedone syndrome'.

ii. This condition is unrelated to the dog's atopy. The syndrome is a disorder of keratinization characterized by dilated cystic hair follicles that develop into comedones. In the author's experience, many dogs have undiagnosed concurrent yeast and bacterial pyodermas associated with this syndrome.

iii. This is a genetic skin disease that can be controlled, but not cured. Owners should be educated not to manipulate the comedones or to scrub the area aggressively, as these dilated hair follicles rupture easily and may become infected. These dogs may have secondary bacterial and yeast infections that are often undiagnosed. Impression smears of the contents of the comedones should be cytologically examined and concurrent infections treated. The hair coat should be kept short to facilitate bathing with a mild shampoo. These dogs require baths 1–3 times per week. Benzoyl peroxide is an excellent follicular flushing shampoo and may be helpful in removing comedones. Antiseborrheic shampoos may also be used. The most important aspect of treatment is to clean the skin without being unduly harsh.

44 One of six beagle puppies, all with similar lesions, was presented for examination. The owner's complaint was that all the dogs had itchy skin and nonhealing 'sores' on the chest, legs, and abdomen. The owner had treated the lesions with topical povidone-iodine scrubs and topical antibiotic ointment with no response. The puppies were being trained to hunt and were housed outside on straw

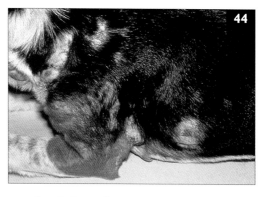

bedding and marsh hay that was removed and changed once or twice monthly. The puppy presented had straw in its hair coat and smelled of feces and urine. Well-demarcated, thickened, hairless lesions with central areas of exudation were present, most notably on the ventral aspect of the dog's body (44).
i. What are the differential diagnoses, and what initial diagnostic tests are indicated?
ii. Skin scrapings revealed nematode larvae about 600 μm in length. What is the diagnosis and treatment?
iii. What other helminth parasites can cause skin disease in dogs and people?

45 A 2-year-old indoor, male, neutered cat was presented for the complaint of symmetrical alopecia due to overgrooming of acute onset (45). This behavior began shortly after the owner remarried; the new spouse had three small children. At the time of examination, it had been occurring for 4 weeks. Skin scrapings, flea combings, and a fungal culture were normal or negative. The owners practiced flea control. A skin biopsy

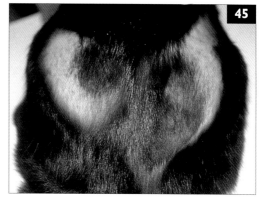

revealed normal skin and hair follicles with no evidence of an inflammatory infiltrate. The cat was normal on physical examination except for growling when the overgroomed site was touched, and palpation of the area revealed pain.
i. What diagnostic test is indicated and why?
ii. What is feline hyperesthesia syndrome, and how is it differentiated clinically from obsessive compulsive grooming?

44, 45: Answers

44 i. The most common pediatric skin diseases are dermatophytosis, louse infestations, fleas, demodicosis, *Sarcoptes*, hookworm dermatitis, and *Pelodera* dermatitis. In this case, demodicosis and secondary deep bacterial infection would be highly suspicious because of the clinical signs. Skin scrapings should be performed to rule out *Demodex* mites and nematodes. Impression smears should be done to look for infectious agents and to confirm the presence of bacterial pyoderma. A dermatophyte culture also should be done; *Microsporum canis* and *M. gypseum* are common dermatophyte infestations of young dogs. Flea combings should be performed to look for macroscopic parasites such as lice and fleas. Sometimes *Cheyletiella* infestations require microscopic confirmation; the mites are small and look like 'moving dandruff'.
ii. *Pelodera* dermatitis (also called rhabditic dermatitis) is caused by a free-living nematode (*Pelodera strongyloides*) found in damp soil, hay, and marsh hay. It invades the skin of dogs housed in filthy conditions and causes severe pruritus. Treatment requires removal of the bedding, cleaning of the facility, bathing of the affected dogs, and antimicrobial therapy for the secondary infections. Parasiticidal dips can be used, but most cases spontaneously resolve once sanitation is improved. Depending upon the severity of the pruritus, humane use of glucocorticoids may be needed to provide relief.
iii. *Ancylostoma braziliense*, *A. caninum*, *Uncinaria stenocephala*, *Gnathostoma spinigerum*, and *Strongyloides stercoralis* have been reported to cause skin disease in people and dogs (Scott *et al.*, 2001a; Smith *et al.*, 1976).

45 i. Radiographs of the caudal abdomen and pelvis are indicated. This is a case of symmetrical alopecia; however, the pattern of overgrooming is somewhat abnormal being asymmetrical and 'curved'. In addition, the cat growling when petted over the area should raise suspicion that the cat is licking the area in response to pain, as opposed to anxiety. Radiographs of the caudal abdomen and pelvis revealed bilateral fractures of the pelvis. After an appropriate period of cage confinement and pain management, the pelvic fractures healed, and the cat's overgrooming stopped. It was eventually discovered that the cat had been run over with a tricycle, and this was presumed to be the cause of the fracture.
ii. Feline hyperesthesia syndrome is not believed to be a behavioral disorder, but rather a disorder of neuropathic pain. Cats affected with this disorder violently groom and self-mutilate themselves in random unpredictable explosive attacks. They often growl, vocalize, run, and may attack others. Owners describe the cats acting as if they are in pain. The skin over the dorsum of the back may twitch or ripple just prior to an episode. In contrast, cats with compulsive grooming behavior show none of the previously described behaviours and methodically groom themselves in secret or in sight.

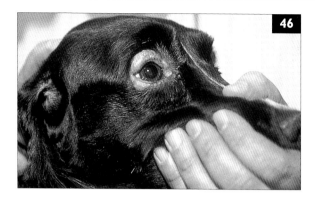

46 A 3-year-old male Labrador retriever dog was presented for acute intermittent episodes of bilateral periocular edema and facial pruritus, a recurrent problem for the last 4 months. The owners reported the dog would be normal for several days, and then acutely develop periocular edema (46). These episodes always happened while the dog was inside the house, in the owner's opinion. What was most frustrating was the episodes would last for several hours, and then the edema would resolve when the dog was taken outside or while en route to the veterinary clinic. After each episode, the dog had some residual periocular or facial pruritus for 1–2 days. The owner was wondering if the lesions were behavioral in origin because they always occurred while she was at home. The owner never arrived home to find the dog with lesions. Conjunctival swabs and aspirates of the edematous area revealed large numbers of eosinophils.

i. What is the clinical diagnosis?
ii. Exposure to some type of allergen is suspected. What questions should the owner be asked, and how might the allergic trigger be identified?
iii. What are the afferent and efferent phases of allergic contact dermatitis?

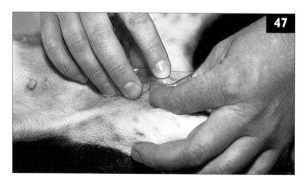

47 What procedure is demonstrated in the illustration (47)?

46 i. Edema is a clinical sign of a type 1 hypersensitivity reaction. The intermittent nature of the episodes suggests some type of allergic reaction, most likely infrequent contact with a potent allergen to which the dog has become sensitized. An underlying allergic etiology is further supported by the presence of eosinophils.

ii. It is difficult to solve cases such as these. The fact that the episodes always happen in the home and not after being outside, suggests that the allergen is located indoors. Also, the intermittent nature of the episodes suggests that the allergen is not present at all times. The final clue is the observation that the owner is always home when the episodes occur. The owner should be asked about the dog's exposure to liquid or aerosol chemicals and cleaning supplies. If there is no obvious cause, the owner should be instructed to keep a log of household activities (cleaning, burning of scented candles, indoor grilling) for several weeks to help to establish a pattern. After careful questioning, reviewing the activity log, and provocative challenge, the dog was found to be developing allergic blepharitis (i.e. allergic contact dermatitis) when the owner used a wood resin for a hobby craft (basket weaving). Improving ventilation and keeping the dog outside when the owner used the wood resin solved the problem. If lesions did develop, the owner was instructed to apply a topical ophthalmic glucocorticoid to the periocular area.

iii. The afferent phase of allergic contact dermatitis is used to describe the initial presentation and processing of the allergen or hapten. The hapten is transferred from the skin to the regional lymph nodes via Langerhans' cells. The stimulated T-lymphocytes produce skin homing ligands that will direct their movement to the skin. The efferent phase describes the animal's response to exposure to the allergen or hapten. After re-exposure to the hapten, activated T-lymphocytes are recruited to the site by expression of adhesion molecules and epidermal cytokines (Belisto, 1999).

47 This is an example of a skin impression smear. The target skin area is gently 'lifted' toward the glass slide to enhance sample collection. The glass microscope slide is then pressed onto the site. In order to obtain a cellular sample, it is very important to apply pressure directly over the target lesion. Using digital pressure from the index finger or thumb easily accomplishes this, minimizing the chance of breaking the glass slide during the impression smear. Enough pressure has been applied if there is an impression of cell debris on the unstained slide. If *Malassezia* is being tested for, the slide should be heat fixed. Care should be taken when heat fixing slides. Matches and butane lighters can leave carbon deposits on the glass slide while a low blue flame from a Bunsen burner will not. If deposits are seen, the material should be gently wiped off the slide prior to examination. Furthermore, heat fixing of glass slides may damage cellular architecture. Thus, at least one slide should be examined without heat fixing.

48 The ventral abdominal area of a 5-year old bull terrier dog is shown (48). The dog lives outside in the state of Colorado, USA, and 'sunbathes' year round in the owner's yard. The lesions depicted include diffuse erythema, several raised erythematous masses, and numerous cutaneous horns. Two years ago, prior to the development of the raised masses, a skin biopsy specimen was obtained. No evidence of neoplasia was seen and the mor-

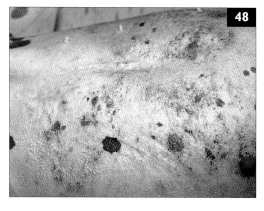

phological diagnosis was 'chronic dermatitis, solar elastosis, and actinic dermatitis/keratoses'. No treatment recommendations were made.

i. What are solar elastosis and actinic dermatitis/keratoses?

ii. What treatment recommendations should have been made?

iii. If a skin biopsy specimen is examined, what is the most likely diagnosis, and what are the treatment recommendations?

49 A cat was presented for the complaint of 'swollen toes' of 3 months' duration (49). Examination revealed generalized paronychia, exudation, and self-trauma on the dorsal skin of the digits. The owner reported that previous skin scrapings were negative for mites and a dermatophyte culture was negative.

i. What diagnostic test(s) should be performed at this time?

ii. Large numbers of neutrophils

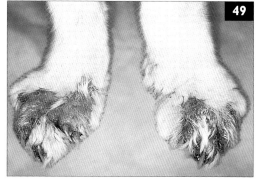

and rare acanthocytes are found on the in-house diagnostic test. How should this case be managed?

iii. Surgical removal of the third phalanx is often required to establish a definitive diagnosis or to rule out suspected differential diagnoses in diseases of the claw. What histological features of normal claws can be mistaken for pathological findings?

48 i. Solar elastosis (damaged elastin fibers in the dermis) and actinic dermatitis (atypia and dysplasia of the epidermis) are terms used to describe skin that has been damaged by excessive exposure to sunlight. Actinic keratoses are crusted hyperkeratotic plaques on the skin; these are premalignant lesions.

ii. The owners should have been advised to keep the dog out of the sunlight, provide photo protection via sunscreens, and/or a canine sun suit. Topical sunscreens labeled as safe for use in infants are recommended, and the highest SPF number available should be used. The owner should have been told to apply sunscreen at least twice a day, clearly before the dog went outside. Topical or oral glucocorticoids could have been used to provide relief from pain or pruritus, if present, and lesions could have been treated with systemic retinoids (isotretinoin, acitretin).

iii. The most likely diagnosis is squamous cell carcinoma. At this stage, surgical excision is unlikely to be curative. These tumors are slow to metastasize, but they are locally invasive. Alternative treatments might include a combination of surgery with radiation therapy, chemotherapy, and photodynamic therapy. Piroxicam, a nonsteroidal anti-inflammatory drug has been used in some dogs in addition to systemic retinoids.

49 i. Impression smears of the nail bed exudates and interdigital exudates should be examined for bacteria and yeast, and a skin biopsy of the nail bed is indicated. Dermatophytosis and PF are the most common causes of paronychia in cats.

ii. Since previous diagnostics ruled out dermatophytosis and mite infestations, the likely causes were a pustular disease such as PF or bacterial pyoderma. The acanthocytes (rounded epithelial cells shed from the stratum spinosum) seen in the cytological specimen were suggestive of pemphigus, as this is a classic finding. However, care must be used when examining slides from deep pyoderma. With severe infection, it is common to see occasional acanthocytes. In PF, rafts of cells are usually found on impression smears of exudate from new lesions. In this case, a practical approach would be to delay any therapy until the biopsy report was received because the problem was of 3 months' duration. However, it was clear from the clinical picture and in-house diagnostics that the lesions were inflamed and exudative. Pending the biopsy report, a course of oral antibiotics (e.g. cephalexin liquid suspension) was prescribed. This was a case of bacterial paronychia, and the cat was almost normal by the time the biopsy report was received.

iii. Intrakeratinocyte vacuoles, intraepidermal and dermoepidermal clefts, pseudo-spongiosis, and apoptotic keratinocytes can be features of normal dog and cat claws, and might be misinterpreted as 'abnormal findings' by a nondermatopathologist (Scott, 2002).

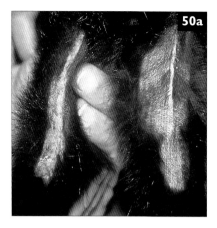

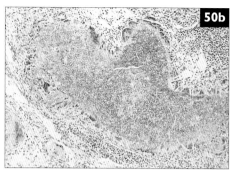

50 An 8-month-old kitten is presented for raised, firm, pencil-like lesions on the caudal aspects of both hind legs. The owner reports the lesions developed rapidly but do not seem bothersome to the kitten. Dermatological examination reveals hard, linear lesions in the superficial dermis (50a). Skin biopsies reveal eosinophilic granulomatous inflammation and collagen degeneration (50b).

i. What is the diagnosis and what are other clinical presentations of the same 'syndrome'?

ii. What are the treatment options?

iii. What components of eosinophil granules may be responsible for collagen degradation?

51 A 10-year-old great Dane dog is presented for evaluation of a mass on the sternum (51). The owner reports that the mass has developed slowly over the last several years. On clinical examination, a raised, freely movable, roughened mass can be found on the sternum. Closer examination of the mass reveals it is a confluent mass of enlarged and dilated hair follicles packed with sebum. Thick black caseous material can be expressed from the pores.

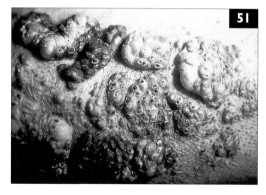

i. What is this lesion called, and how should it be treated?

ii. What is a hygroma, and how is it managed?

iii. What is a 'tug of war blister'?

50 i. This is a classic presentation of feline eosinophilic granuloma. Other presentations include firm swellings on the chin (fat chin syndrome), swollen lower lips (pouting cat syndrome), oral lesions in the mouth, firm nodules in the skin, and nodules on the ear pinnae.

ii. Treatment is not always needed as lesions in cats less than 1 year of age usually spontaneously resolve. Methylprednisone acetate (20 mg/cat SC), every 2 weeks until the lesions resolve (4–6 weeks), is effective. Recurrent lesions suggest an underlying trigger such as FAD, food allergy, and/or atopy.

iii. The pathogenesis of these lesions is unknown. However, tissue damage may be caused by eosinophil collagenase that degrades type I and II collagen and gelatinases that degrade type XVII collagen.

51 i. This is a sternal callus, and it is a type of pressure point injury caused by repeated trauma to skin. The skin and specialized structures have proliferated resulting in the development of cystic comedones and furunculosis. These lesions are difficult to treat because they tend to recur. In this case, the area should be hot packed and gently washed daily with benzoyl peroxide. If there is limited fibrosis, it may be possible to massage gently the lesion with a circular motion and express the black debris from the comedones. Extreme care must be taken not to be aggressive as this may result in further rupture of hair follicles. Concurrent systemic antibiotics for 4–6 weeks are helpful. It is unlikely that this lesion will completely resolve because of its severity and chronicity. Surgical excision would be difficult due to concerns about wound closure. In addition to medical management, the dog should sleep on a soft padded bed; many dogs with this condition elect to sleep on hard surfaces even when provided with soft bed options.

ii. A hygroma is a false bursa that occurs over bony prominences and pressure points, especially in large breed dogs. Repeated trauma from lying on hard surfaces produces an inflammatory response, which results in a dense-walled, fluid-filled cavity. A soft, fluctuant (fluid-filled), painless swelling develops over pressure points, especially the olecranon. If long-standing, severe inflammation may develop, and ulceration, infection, abscesses, granulomas, and fistulas may develop. The bursa contains a clear, yellow to red fluid. If diagnosed early and if still small, hygromas can be managed medically via aseptic needle aspiration, followed by corrective housing. Soft bedding or padding over pressure points is imperative to prevent further trauma. If hygromas are chronic, surgical drainage, flushing, and placement of Penrose drains are indicated. Areas with severe ulceration may require extensive drainage, extirpation, or skin grafting procedures. Use of intrahygromal corticosteroids is not recommended.

iii. A 'tug of war blister' (Scott *et al.*, 2001c) is a traumatic injury characterized by vesicles and erosions on the front paws of dogs that vigorously play 'tug of war'. Lesions have an acute onset in an otherwise healthy dog. These lesions may be more common in puppies where pads are more fragile or in breeds of dogs with a high threshold of pain.

52 A 1-year-old female indoor cat from Florida was presented for an after-hours emergency examination. Approximately 72 hours after spending the night locked out on the family's screened-in porch, the cat developed acute severe facial pruritus and was presented for the lesions shown (52). Similar lesions were seen on the ear tips and paws; only thinly haired areas with dark hair were affected. The cat was otherwise healthy. Skin scrapings were negative. Impression smears of

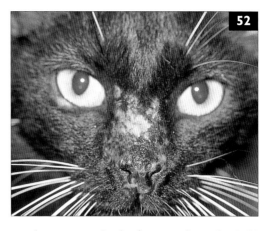

the nose revealed inflammatory exudates comprised of approximately 75% eosinophils and lesser numbers of neutrophils, lymphocytes, and mast cells.

i. This cat's lesions are most compatible with what differential diagnoses? Based upon the information provided, what is the most likely diagnosis?

ii. The owners declined a skin biopsy. How would the likely disease then be confirmed? What are the treatment recommendations?

iii. What would be expected on a skin biopsy specimen from this cat?

53 A Labrador retriever dog was presented for examination because the dog had a 'pink nose' (53). The owner reported that the dog's nose and skin were normal until several months ago. At that time, she noticed a small amount of crusting at the junction of the haired and unhaired regions of the nose. When this crusting sloughed, the lesion depicted was present. The owner reported that sometimes crusting is present in this area, but she removes it as soon as it develops. No other abnormalities were found on examination.

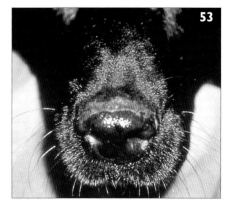

i. What condition is seen here, what are the differential diagnoses, and what diagnostic test(s) is/are most cost effective in making a definitive diagnosis?

ii. What is the most common cause of hypopigmentation in dogs?

iii. List five hereditary causes of hypopigmentation that have been documented in dogs or cats.

52, 53: Answers

52 i. PF or pemphigus erythematosus, food allergy, atopy, dermatophytosis, and insect bite hypersensitivity. The most likely diagnosis is insect bite hypersensitivity, particularly mosquito-bite hypersensitivity. The clinical lesions and history are characteristic of the disease. The rapid development of the lesions after spending the night outside (most screened porches are not insect proof) and the marked eosinophilia seen on cytological examination of impression smears are highly supportive of the diagnosis. Mosquitoes are attracted to dark colors or dark hair coats; lesions are often seen in the darkly haired areas of cats.

ii. This disease is seasonal and coincides with the mosquito season, although other small biting insects (gnats, *Culicoides* spp.) can cause similar lesions. Confining the cat indoors for 5–7 days and watching for lesion resolution can confirm the diagnosis; the other differential diagnoses will not respond to this therapy. Keeping the cat indoors can prevent recurrences. Also, improving the quality of the screening and/or using a flea control product with repellant activity is recommended. Permethrins can be toxic to cats, and only products labeled as safe for use in cats should be used. Dimethyl metatolulimide (DEET) should not be used in cats. Repositol methylprednisolone 5 mg/kg subcutaneously may be needed to resolve lesions and/or treat cats that cannot be confined. This therapy is safe if the problem is seasonal. This cat was treated with one injection of methylprednisolone (20 mg/cat SC) and the lesions resolved within 14 days. The lesions recurred if the cat spent excessive time on the family's screened porch in the evening when mosquitoes were present.

iii. Histological findings most compatible with this syndrome include a superficial and deep eosinophilic infiltrate. Unique findings in this disease include infiltrative eosinophilic mural folliculitis and furunculosis, dermal mucinosis, and flame figures. Such skin biopsy findings are relatively common in arthropod or insect bites.

53 i. Nasal hypopigmentation or nasal depigmentation. Note the depigmentation on the dorsum of the nose at the junction of the haired and unhaired skin of the nose. Also, note the subtle depigmentation of the nares. Differential diagnoses include discoid lupus erythematosus, trauma, contact allergy (rare), pemphigus complex, and cutaneous lymphoma. A skin biopsy of the depigmented area and nares is the most cost effective diagnostic test. In cases of nasal hypopigmentation, skin biopsy specimens should be obtained from the oldest (i.e. most depigmented or gray area). This was a case of lupus erythematosus.

ii. The most common cause of hypopigmentation in dogs is graying of the hair as a result of senescence of melanocytes.

iii. Chediak–Higashi syndrome in Persian cats, albinism, piebaldism, Warrdenburg–Klein syndrome, and canine cyclic hematopoiesis of collie dogs.

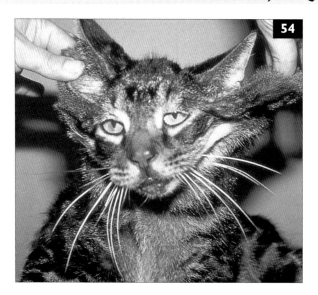

54 A 5-year-old male cat with classical signs of a heritable skin disease is shown (54).
i. What is the diagnosis?
ii. What other clinical signs are associated with this disorder, how is this disease treated and, excluding euthanasia, what is the most common cause of death in these cats?
iii. What is the biochemical cause of this disease?

55 This cat was diagnosed with what was previously called 'feline endocrine alopecia' (55).
i. What is the hormonal abnormality of feline endocrine alopecia?
ii. What is the current terminology for this condition?
iii. What are the most common differential diagnoses for this disorder?

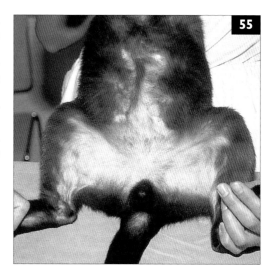

54, 55: Answers

54 i. Ehlers–Danlos syndrome, cutaneous asthenia, or dermatosparaxis. This disease can occur in both dogs and cats.
ii. The skin is soft, pliable, 'stretchy', and loosely attached to the underlying epidermis. These cats will often present with nonhealing wounds, bleeding, and tears from minimal trauma. Some animals have joint laxity and/or ocular changes, and clinical signs often worsen with age. This is a hereditary disease, and affected animals should not be bred from. There is no known treatment. Pets with mild symptoms and/or joint laxity may be kept as pets; however, most are eventually euthanized because of the recurrent skin tears. Affected cats may die suddenly from rupture of an aortic aneurysm or other large vessel.
iii. This is an inherited disease caused by a biochemical defect in collagen production. Affected collagen forms twisted ribbons rather than cylindric fibrils and fibers. Biochemical studies have demonstrated a procollagen production defect, resulting in decreased activity of procollagen peptidase, and accumulation of partially processed type I procollagen containing N-terminal propeptides. Collagenase activity is increased several-fold above normal (Minor, 1987; Scott *et al.*, 2001e).

55 i. Feline endocrine alopecia is a misnomer, and there is no hormonal abnormality in these cats.
ii. The current terminology for this condition is FSA.
iii. FSA is a dermatological reaction pattern caused by a wide range of feline skin diseases. The hair loss is caused by overgrooming. Less commonly, it can be a clinical manifestation of obsessive-compulsive behavior in cats. The standard evaluation of these cats is to rule out parasitic, infectious, and allergic skin diseases prior to making a diagnosis of psychogenic alopecia. Skin scrapings, flea combings, acetate tape preparations, fecal examinations, and treatment trials with ivermectin and/or flea control should be performed to rule out parasites. Dermatophyte cultures and impression smears for bacteria and *Malassezia* dermatitis should be obtained to rule out infectious agents.

If bacterial or yeast dermatitis is found, then a careful search for the underlying trigger is necessary while the infections are treated. Food allergy, flea allergy, and atopy should be ruled out via food trials, flea control trials, and skin testing, and/or *in vitro* allergy testing, respectively. Finally, a skin biopsy should be performed to rule out inflammatory infiltrates in the skin. A complete blood count to look for signs of infection and/or eosinophilia may be helpful. An elevated eosinophil count is often seen in cats with fleas and/or FAD. If the cat is older, a complete serum chemistry panel, thyroid hormone evaluation, and urinalysis should be done to rule out systemic illnesses as a cause of FSA. Diseases such as feline hyperthyroidism, diabetes mellitus, chronic renal disease, and neoplasia should be considered as possible metabolic diseases associated with FSA.

56 The medial thigh of a dog scheduled for surgery for repair of a ruptured anterior cruciate ligament is shown (56). As part of the pre-operative procedures, the dog was bathed in an antibacterial shampoo (benzoyl peroxide), and then given an intravenous bolus of a second-generation cephalosporin. A student bathed the dog in a stainless steel tub in warm water and then towel dried the dog. Approximately 20 minutes later, the dog had a generalized eruption of coalescing erythematous wheals. The dog was pruritic, but showed no gastrointestinal symptoms.

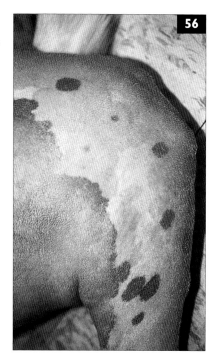

i. What is the most likely diagnosis?
ii. What caused the reaction seen, and how should this patient be treated?
iii. What is/are the mechanisms involved in the development of these lesions?

57 A bacterial culture and sensitivity is performed on a dog with recurrent bacterial pyoderma. The laboratory isolates *Staphylococcus intermedius* and reports that the organism is sensitive to the following drugs:
- Tetracycline.
- Penicillin.
- Amoxicillin.
- Cephalosporin.
- Chloramphenicol.
- Erythromycin.
- Sulfonamide.
- Amoxicillin clavulanate.
- Enrofloxacin.

i. Which of these drugs are least likely to be efficacious in the treatment of canine pyoderma even though the sensitivity shows susceptibility?
ii. Which of these drugs, although effective against *S. intermedius*, is best avoided for the treatment of canine pyoderma?

56 i. The erythematous wheals are classic for urticaria, which is a type 1 hyper-sensitivity reaction. Folliculitis, vasculitis, erythema multiforme, and neoplasia can also mimic urticarial lesions, but the sudden occurrence of the lesions in this case makes these differential diagnoses unlikely.

ii. Type 1 hypersensitivity reactions, such as urticaria, usually occur within 1 hour of exposure to the offending allergen. In this patient, the urticarial reactions could have been caused by any one of the shampoo ingredients (coloring, scent, benzoyl peroxide, detergent agents), the antibiotic (drug, carrier agent), the water temperature, the pressure from towel drying the patient, or the disinfectant used to clean the bathing tub or the dog's run. It is also possible that it was a combination of factors that led to the eruption.

This patient was closely monitored for signs of systemic anaphylaxis (vomiting and diarrhea), immediately bathed with water to remove any shampoo residue, and given prednisone (2 mg/kg IM). Epinephrine was not administered because the dog did not show signs of systemic anaphylaxis. If he had, epinephrine (1:1000 in 0.1–0.5 ml SC or IM) in addition to prednisone would have been administered. Antihistamines were not used because they are ineffective in the treatment of acute episodes of urticaria even though they are beneficial in preventing future reactions. Finally, the surgeon elected not to use cephalosporin antibiotics in this patient.

Interestingly, follow-up of this patient revealed that he had a history of recurrent episodes of urticaria associated with stressful events (car rides, visits to the veterinarian's office, boarding in a kennel). Pre-treatment with an antihistamine (hydroxyzine 2 mg/kg PO q8h) before these events eliminated the problem.

iii. Urticaria and angioedema can result from immunological and nonimmunological mast cell or basophil degranulation. Increased vascular permeability causes extra-vasculation of fluid into the tissues. Immunological mechanisms involve type 1 and type 3 reactions. Nonimmunological mechanisms include physical forces (heat, sunlight, cold, exercise, pressure), psychological stresses, genetic abnormalities, drugs, and chemicals.

57 i. Tetracycline, penicillin, and amoxicillin are generally best avoided in the treat-ment of canine pyoderma. Although the sensitivity in this case shows that the organism is sensitive, the clinical response in patients treated with these drugs is often poor.

ii. Enrofloxacin, a fluoroquinolone, is best avoided in the routine treatment of canine pyoderma. There are other less expensive and equally efficacious drugs. Another important reason to avoid the routine use of fluoroquinolone antibiotics in the treatment of bacterial pyoderma is the concern over the development of resistant bacterial strains. This is particularly true in the case of *Pseudomonas*.

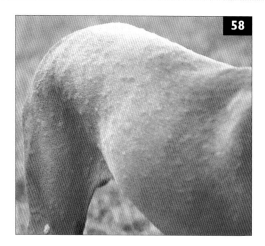

58 A 7-month-old dog was presented for the first time for the complaint of 'bumps', a common clinical presentation of superficial bacterial pyoderma in dogs (58). Note the 'goose bump' or 'hive'-like lesions on the skin.

i. What is the name of this condition, and what is seen upon close examination of the skin?

ii. What differential diagnoses and diagnostic tests should be performed to confirm the diagnosis?

iii. What is the mechanism of action of fluoroquinolone antibiotics, and why would this drug class not be an appropriate antibiotic choice in this dog?

59 An impression smear from the nail bed debris from a dog with intense pedal pruritus is shown (59).

i. What is this organism, and how do dogs contract it?

ii. What species have been isolated from dogs and cats?

iii. Is this a zoonosis?

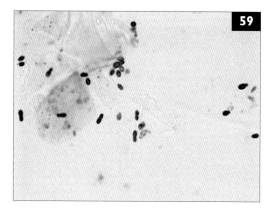

58 i. This is an example of superficial bacterial infection of the skin involving the hair follicles, hence the name 'superficial bacterial folliculitis'. Close examination of the skin revealed small papules at the base of the hairs. These papules/pustules may rupture causing the formation of tiny epidermal collarettes, which may be seen encircling the base of the hairs.

ii. The major differential diagnoses to consider are: dermatophytosis, demodicosis, and *Malassezia* dermatitis. Less common differential diagnoses include pemphigus, sterile eosinophilic pustulosis, and pustular demodicosis. Most commonly, however, bacterial folliculitis is likely to be confused with dermatophytosis or urticaria. Skin scrapings should be performed to rule out demodicosis, impression smears to rule out concurrent *Malassezia* infections, and dermatophyte cultures where there is a suspicion of infection.

The diagnosis of a bacterial pyoderma is often a clinical diagnosis supported by ruling out demodicosis and dermatophytosis, the two most common follicular diseases. Concurrent bacterial and *Malassezia* infections, especially in warm weather, can occur in approximately 50% of patients.

iii. Fluoroquinolone antibiotics act intracellularly by preventing bacterial DNA synthesis by partly inhibiting bacterial DNA gyrase. This class of drugs is primarily active against Gram-negative aerobic and facultative anaerobic bacteria. Although they are effective against many Gram-positive organisms (e.g. staphylococci), the minimum inhibitory concentrations are usually higher than for Gram-negative bacteria. Fluoroquinolone antibiotics are contraindicated in this particular patient because they are known to cause an erosive arthropathy in young dogs.

59 i. *Malassezia* spp. *Malassezia* organisms are part of the normal fungal flora of the skin of dogs, and they have been isolated from 3-day-old puppies. Their resident niche is the oral cavity, ears, anal sacs, interdigital areas, and mucocutaneous junctions. These organisms can also be found on the skin of normal dogs, but not easily and not in large numbers. Controversy exists as to 'how many organisms' are too many. In the author's opinion, if the animal is symptomatic and organisms are found, treatment is indicated.

ii. *Malassezia pachydermatitis* is the only species isolated from dogs. *M. pachydermatitis*, *M. sympodialis*, and *M. globosa* have been isolated from cats.

iii. *M. pachydermatitis* can transiently colonize the skin of people. It was the presumed cause of an outbreak of exfoliative dermatitis, septicemia, meningitis, and urinary tract infections in a neonatal intensive care unit. The organism was then transferred from human to human in the unit.

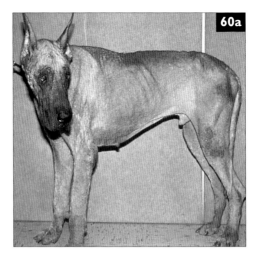

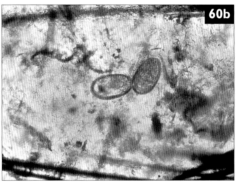

60 This great Dane dog was presented for examination. It was one of 12 dogs in a kennel, all of which had had intense pruritus for 1 year (60a). The owners reported that the other dogs looked similar to this one. In addition to skin lesions, the dogs were losing weight and were irritable with the owners and each other. Close examination of the skin revealed a generalized papular eruption without evidence of pustules and/or epidermal collarettes. Any manipulation of the skin triggered an intense episode of self-mutilation. All of the dogs were currently vaccinated, received monthly heartworm medication, and monthly spot-on flea control. The owners reported no lesions or discomfort after any handling of the dogs. Flea combings were negative. Skin scrapings revealed the organism shown (60b).

i. What is the diagnosis?

ii. The owners of the kennel have three border collie dogs and seven cats in addition to these dogs. What are the treatment options for this kennel of dogs? What is the cause and what treatment can be used for cat scabies?

60 i. Scabies infestation. The organism is an egg of *Sarcoptes* spp. One mite or egg is diagnostic for scabies. Definitive evidence of a scabies infestation (eggs or mites) is not always found, even in 'classic cases'. The vast majority of dogs with scabies are diagnosed based upon response to treatment, hence the old saying with regard to scabies in dogs: 'If you suspect it, treat for it'.

ii. Scabies mites can live for a short period of time off the host. The kennel facilities should be thoroughly cleaned with high-pressure hoses, scrubbed with detergent, and then sprayed with an environmental parasiticidal agent. Any and all dogs in contact with these great Dane dogs should be treated for scabies. Lime sulfur dips once weekly for 6 weeks or amitraz dips every 2 weeks for 6 weeks are effective topical therapies. Lime sulfur can be combined with ivermectin therapy. Ivermectin (200 µg/kg PO or SC) every 2 weeks for 6 weeks is also a very effective treatment. The author uses a test dose of 100 µg/kg PO in all dogs. If there are no adverse effects consistent with ivermectin sensitivity (e.g. tremors, salivation) within 24 hours, a full treatment dose of 200 µg/kg PO is administered the next day.

Herding breeds of dogs, especially collies, are known to be sensitive to ivermectin toxicity. Thus, the drug is best avoided in this breed. Dogs sensitive to ivermectin can often tolerate milbemycin oxime at 3 mg/kg PO weekly for 3–6 weeks. Lime sulfur dips are also an effective therapy. Doramectin at 0.2 mg/kg SC or IM has also been reported to be effective. Finally, two applications of selamectin or fipronil at 30 day intervals may be effective. Selamectin is licensed for the treatment of scabies, and the manufacturer reported it to be effective in 70% of cases. Fipronil is not licensed for use but has been found to be effective. Again the author has seen treatment failure cases with this drug. It is important to remember that no one treatment is 100% efficacious in all patients. If scabies is suspected and the patient does not respond, retreatment with a different therapy should be performed before ruling it out.

Canine scabies is not considered a contagion to cats. However, *Sarcoptes* mites have been reported in a small number of cats with severe debilitation and in pruritic cats in England. There may be some geographic variation with respect to contagion to cats. These cats do not need to be treated. True 'feline scabies' is caused by *Notoedres cati*, a contagious mange mite. In contrast to canine scabies, *N. cati* is easily found in large numbers on skin scrapings. In cats, lesions are found on the head, feet, and perineum. This infestation can cause large amounts of crust; cats should be sedated, the hair coat clipped, and the cat bathed to remove the contaminated crusts prior to treatment. Because cats are extremely sensitive to parasiticidal agents, lime sulfur and ivermectin are the most commonly used treatments. Affected cats, and all animals in contact with infection should be treated for at least 6 weeks.

61 A cat was found as a stray in winter in Wisconsin, USA, during a January blizzard. The cat was suffering from hypothermia and had frostbite on the ear margins, tail tip, and on several digits. The cat recovered from the hypothermia and the only permanent damage was sloughing of the tail tip, several digits, and the tips of the ears, the latter healing with a slightly irregular contour. Over the last 5 years, the cat has been

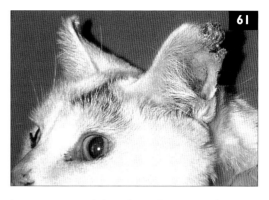

an indoor cat. Several months ago, the owners noted that the cat's ear margins were crusted and bleeding (61).

i. What is the most likely differential diagnosis?

ii. What role, if any, did the frostbite have in the development of the lesions? At this time, what is the most cost effective treatment?

iii. What is Bowen's disease?

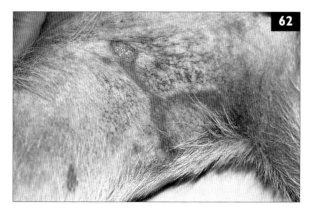

62 The inguinal fold area of a partially paralyzed dog is shown (62). The dog was expected to regain voluntary movement and was released to the owners for home care. The owners manually expressed the dog's bladder six times per day; however, the dog was often found wet from urine leakage.

i. What is the most likely cause of the lesion shown?

ii. How should this lesion be treated to prevent it from happening again?

iii. What are the most common irritants encountered by small animals?

61 i. This is a white cat with lesions on the ear margins. The most likely cause is squamous cell carcinoma. Many cats with squamous cell carcinomas will have pre-cancerous actinic changes of the skin prior to the development of the lesion. Actinic skin changes are most commonly seen in the external ear pinnae and pre-auricular areas. Owners may report a waxing and waning of erythema and scaling in these areas.

ii. Frostbite, though uncommon in animals, usually affects the tips of the ears. Healing is slow, and as the necrotic tissue sloughs, the remaining ear margins will curl. Ear margins are notorious for healing slowly due to poor vascularization. Because squamous cell carcinomas have been observed to develop at the site of frostbite scars in people, it is possible that frostbite predisposed this cat to squamous cell carcinoma. The most cost effective therapy is bilateral pinnectomy. This was a case of bilateral squamous cell carcinoma in a cat. These tumors have low metastatic rates, and radical, local therapy can result in a long-term cure. Although surgical excision of the ears seemed rather 'dramatic' to the owner, the surgeon was able to obtain clean margins, and the lesions did not recur. In addition to surgery, minimizing sun exposure was recommended, a nearly impossible task in this species.

iii. Bowen's disease is also known as multifocal squamous cell carcinoma in situ. This disease can occur in cats or dogs, but is most common in middle-aged cats. In this disorder, multiple squamous cell carcinomas are present in the haired or pigmented skin in a cluster. The lesions are 0.5–4.0 cm in size and may have 1–3 mm of crusts that reveal an ulcer underneath when removed. In cats, these lesions can occur as gingivitis or plaques. The treatment of choice is surgical excision.

62 i. The most likely cause is urine scalding. This is an irritant reaction caused by the skin being chronically wet from exposure to urine.

ii. These lesions are very painful. The area should be washed with warm water and thoroughly dried. Topical silver sulfadiazine ointment or triple antibiotic ointment should be applied to this lesion until it heals. Urine scald lesions are a risk factor in any animal that is recumbent and/or paralyzed. The owners need to express the dog's bladder more efficiently and/or more frequently. If this dog is having urine scalding, it is very likely that the dog may also develop pressure point necrosis. The dog should be turned more frequently and consideration should be given to putting the dog in a body sling until it recovers.

iii. Irritant reactions are most likely to occur on thinly haired areas. The most commonly incriminated irritants include soaps, detergents, disinfectants, weed and insecticidal sprays, flea collars, fertilizers, and carpet cleaners or fresheners.

63 A 4-year-old female spayed black Labrador retriever dog was presented for recurrent otitis externa. Dermatological examination was normal except for bilaterally erythematous lacey hyper-pigmentation of the external ear canal and inner pinnae (63a). Otoscopic exam-ination revealed the erythema was limited to the vertical ear canal, and cytological examination using ear swabs revealed numerous keratinocytes and rare *Malassezia* organisms. The dog's otitis responded to topical glucocorticoids, and a working diagnosis of allergic otitis externa was made. Over the next year, the dog developed pedal and facial pruritus. The pruritus continued year round but was worse in the summer and fall. The dog's symptoms were not easily controlled with antihistamines and essential fatty acids. An intradermal skin test was performed and numerous positive reactions were found (63b).

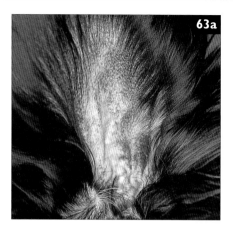

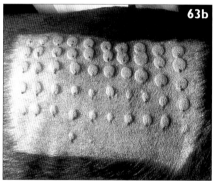

i. What question does an intradermal skin test answer?
ii. How will antigens to include in an immunotherapy mixture be selected?

64 Antibiotic therapy is commonly used in veterinary dermatology. In many diseases it is necessary to obtain a bacterial culture and sensitivity to determine appropriate drug therapy. There are two methods for determining bacterial sensitivity to an organism: disc diffusion and tube dilution.
i. What is the difference between these two tests?
ii. Laboratories using tube dilution tests report an 'MIC numerical value' and identify the organism as S (susceptible), I (intermediately susceptible) and R (resistant). Why does the laboratory report a numerical MIC and why does the laboratory also interpret the susceptibility for the clinician?

63 i. An intradermal skin test does not answer the question of whether or not the patient is atopic. That question is answered by the patient's history, clinical signs, and by ruling out other causes of pruritus. Positive intradermal skin test reactions can provide corroborating support for a diagnosis; however, the major question that needs to be answered is 'what allergens are significant for this patient?' In other words, positive reactions show exposure. Intradermal skin testing and *in vitro* allergy testing are primarily used to guide selection of allergens for immunotherapy. If a client is unwilling to consider immunotherapy, then the cost effectiveness of doing an intradermal skin test or *in vitro* allergy test must be considered.

ii. There are two major criteria for selection of allergens for an immunotherapy mixture. The first is the match between the positive reactions and the patient's symptoms. The second is the strength of the reaction. Allergens are selected for immunotherapy based upon matching the patient's clinical signs to the results of the intradermal skin test. For example, if the patient were not symptomatic in the spring when trees were pollinating, then tree allergens would not be included in immunotherapy mixture. The second criterion takes into consideration the strength or weakness of the intradermal skin test reaction. By convention, intradermal skin test reactions are scored subjectively on a 0–4 scale using wheal size, induration, and erythema; positive and negative controls are used as reference points. Generally, intradermal skin test reactions scoring 2 or greater are considered significant if they correlate with the patient's history.

64 i. The disc diffusion technique is semiquantitative and the drug concentrations in the agar surrounding the disc are roughly proportional to the drug concentrations in the patient's serum. The tube dilution technique is a quantitative method for determining bacterial sensitivity. This technique provides quantitative data regarding the amount of drug required to inhibit bacterial growth. This technique allows for a MIC to be determined by growing bacteria in decreasing concentrations of drug.

ii. Laboratories using the tube dilution technique report a numerical MIC and the more familiar 'S' (susceptible), 'I' (intermediately susceptible) and 'R' (resistant) designations. MIC values are specific to the bacteria cultured and specific drug tested. The designation of S, I, or R relates to the 'breakpoint' MIC. The breakpoint MIC for a specific organism will vary among species. The breakpoint MIC is the highest drug concentration that can be achieved safely with clinically acceptable drug doses and routes of administration. With MIC testing, bacteria are considered to be sensitive to the drug if the MIC is well below the breakpoint MIC. Bacteria are considered to be intermediately susceptible if the MIC approaches the breakpoint MIC and are considered to be resistant if the MIC surpasses the breakpoint.

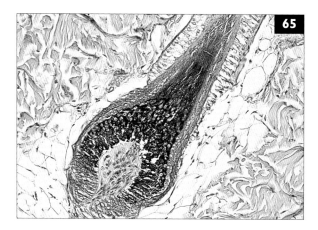

65 A photomicrograph of a cross section of a hair bulb is shown (65).
i. What are the stages of the hair cycle, and what are the most common patterns of growth in dogs and cats?
ii. What factors influence hair growth in animals?
iii. Describe the basic anatomy of a hair follicle.

66 A 9-month-old boxer cross dog is presented for examination of its chin. The owners report that the dog develops 'pimples' in this area. Upon physical examination, the dog has hair loss, papules, and furuncles on the lips, chin, and muzzle (66). Many of the hair follicles are plugged with keratin, and purulent material and hairs can be expressed from within these follicles.
i. What is the common name for this condition?
ii. How is this treated?

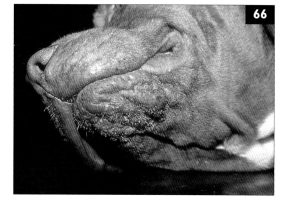

65 i. There are three stages or cycles in hair growth. The first is anagen, or the growing phase. During this time the hair follicle is actively producing hair. The anagen hair is characterized by a well-developed dermal papilla that is covered or 'capped' by the hair matrix. The second stage is catagen, or a transition stage between active growth and rest. This hair is characterized by retraction toward the surface. The catagen hair follicle is shortened in length and smaller. The most characteristic feature of a catagen hair is the replacement of inner root sheath by trichilemmal keratinization. During telogen, or the resting stage, the hair stops growing and is retained in the hair follicle as a dead hair. A telogen hair is characterized as a small hair, approximately one-third the length of the anagen hair. Hairs continue to grow until they reach a preset length and then enter the resting phase. The hair will remain in this state until a new hair starts to grow, pushes the old hair out, and the old hair is shed. Hairs in dogs and cats are replaced in a mosaic pattern with peaks of hair loss/replacement in the spring and fall. The other two most common replacement patterns are seasonal and waves.

ii. The hair cycle of animals is controlled by a number of factors including: photoperiod, ambient temperature, health, genetics (i.e. breed and species), nutrition, hormones, and local factors that directly influence the growth of hair follicles. The most important of these factors are photoperiod and ambient temperature.

iii. Hair follicles are divided into three major anatomical regions: the infundibulum, isthmus, and the inferior segment. The infundibulum or pilosebaceous region consists of the area from the opening of the sebaceous duct to the surface of the skin. The isthmus consists of the area between the opening of the sebaceous duct and the attachment of the arrector pili muscle. The inferior segment extends from the attachment of the arrector pili muscle to the dermal hair papilla.

66 i. 'Canine chin acne' is the common name for this disorder although this is incorrect. 'Acne' is a disorder of keratinization, and the condition depicted is, in reality, a deep furunculosis. Chin furunculosis is almost exclusively seen in short coated dogs such as boxers, doberman pinschers, English bulldogs, great Dane dogs, rottweilers, and German shorthaired pointers. The cause of this condition is unknown, and it is speculated there may be a breed and/or inherited predisposition to the development of muzzle folliculitis and furunculosis.

ii. In young dogs, it is important to rule out demodicosis as an underlying cause or complication of muzzle folliculitis and furunculosis. This condition is treated with oral antibiotics for 4–6 weeks along with daily cleansing of the lesions. It is important to treat the condition aggressively as these lesions can cause scarring.

67 A 4-month-old kitten is presented for evaluation of a freely movable, firm, well-circumscribed, 0.5 cm dermal nodule between the scapulae on the dorsal back. The kitten has a history of being vaccinated 14 days ago in this region. The kitten also has a history of flea and tick infestation.
i. What are the most likely differential diagnoses?
ii. How should the clinician proceed?

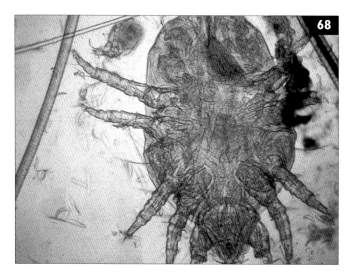

68 The owner of a dog brought in a small container filled with scales. The organism shown was found in the debris (68). What is it, what clinical signs can it cause, and how is it usually diagnosed?

67, 68: Answers

67 i. Injection site reaction, tick bite reaction (tick bite hypersensitivity or tick bite granuloma), focal eosinophilic granuloma. Injection site granuloma is most likely due to recent history of vaccination; however, these clinical diseases cannot easily be differentiated by clinical presentation and history alone. Cats frequently develop local reactions at the site of vaccinations and/or injections. A post-vaccinal fibrosarcoma is unlikely due to the rapid development of this nodule and its clinical presentation (well-circumscribed, freely movable nodule). Post-vaccinal fibrosarcomas occur in subcutaneous tissue at the site of previous injections. These neoplasms tend to be irregular and nodular in shape, soft to firm, poorly circumscribed, and variably sized (1–15 cm). These lesions are often ulcerated and hairless. Feline fibrosarcomas associated with feline sarcoma virus are seen in cats less than 5 years of age and tend to be multicentric.

ii. There are several options available. The first option is surgical excision of the lesion and histological examination of the tissue. The second option would be FNA. Cytological findings in a fibrosarcoma include pleomorphic, atypical fibroblasts. FNA of firm dermal nodules due to granulomatous reactions are difficult to perform and are often poorly cellular; eosinophils and macrophages may be seen. The third option is to measure the lesion and watch it for further development. Tick bite granulomas and injection site reactions are usually maximally developed by the time the owner finds them; these lesions will spontaneously resolve over several weeks. Eosinophilic granulomas may progress, or not. If the lesion progresses, it should be biopsied.

68 This is a *Cheyletiella* spp. mite also called the 'walking dandruff mite'. This mite lives in the superficial layers of the epidermis; it does not burrow. It lays its eggs on hair shafts, and the eggs are smaller and more loosely attached than louse eggs. This is a contagious mange mite that causes scaling and mild to moderate pruritus in contrast to scabies, which causes intense pruritus. In some breeds of dogs (e.g. cocker spaniels), the only clinical sign is excessive scaling that resembles idiopathic seborrhea. This mite can cause skin disease in cats, dogs, and rabbits. It causes scaling, pruritus, miliary dermatitis or, surprisingly, no symptoms in cats. Diagnosis can be difficult because infestations can vary from mild to severe. Mites can be found on skin scrapings, acetate tape preparations, flea combings, and in cats via fecal examination (cats ingest the mites during grooming). In some situations, mites cannot be demonstrated, but animals are pruritic and the owners have clinical lesions consistent with cheyletiellosis. (See also 69.)

69 With regard to the dog in **68** infested with *Cheyletiella* mites:
i. How is this condition treated, and what are the zoonotic implications?
ii. How would this mite be differentiated from others?

70 A 4-year-old dachshund dog is presented for the complaint of recurrent bacterial pyoderma, pruritus, seborrhea, and hair loss in the lumbosacral area (**70a**). The owners are breeders and have been referred for an intradermal skin test for the dog. The episodes of recurrent bacterial pyoderma and seborrhea respond to antibiotic therapy and antiseborrheic shampoo therapy. Physical examination reveals a quiet, slightly overweight dog with bilaterally symmetrical hair loss in the lumbosacral area. The skin of the ventral neck, axilla, inguinal regions, and legs is thickened and folded (**70b**).

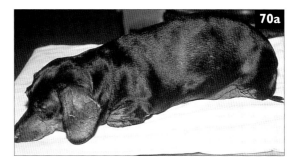
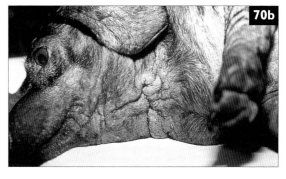

Lichenification, hyperpigmentation, waxy debris, odor, hair loss, and a papular eruption are present. Upon further questioning of the owners, it is established that the dog is not pruritic when the bacterial pyoderma and seborrhea are resolved. Skin scrapings and fungal culture are negative. Impression smears today reveal bacteria and *Malassezia* organisms. During the entire examination, the dog has not moved on the examination table. When this is mentioned to the owners, they respond by saying that they selectively breed for a quiet temperament.

i. Is an intradermal skin test indicated in this patient? Why or why not?
ii. What skin disease(s) may the breeders be inadvertently selecting for in this line of dogs?
iii. The diagnostic suspicions are confirmed. What advice should the clients be offered?

69, 70: Answers

69 i. All animals in contact with an infested host or suspected infested host should be treated. This mite is particularly difficult to eliminate in hosts with long hair, and clipping of the hair coat is strongly recommended. Prior to specific antiparasiticidal treatment, the affected host should be bathed in a flea shampoo to aid in the mechanical removal of mites and eggs. It is very important to treat for at least 4 weeks since the life cycle of the host is 3 weeks. Topical pyrethrin sprays, fipronil spot-on repeated twice at 30 day intervals, fipronil spray, lime sulfur dips weekly for 6 weeks, amitraz sponge-on dips, and milbemycin are effective. Because mites live on the surface of the skin and lay eggs on the hairs, reinfestation or inadequate eradication is very possible if treatment is too short. Furthermore, these mites can live off the host for at least 10 days. The environment should be thoroughly cleaned, and an environmental flea control product should be used to kill mites in areas that the host frequents (dog beds). It is a zoonotic disease, and in many cases owners will report pruritic red papules on their arms, abdomen, and legs or any other area in contact with affected hosts.

ii. *Otodectes* mites are large, white, and move freely on the skin. They are most likely to be found in or near the ears. The anus is terminal, and they have four legs that extend beyond the body wall, except for the 4th pair in females, with short, unjointed stalks with suckers on all four legs in males and the first two pairs in females. *Sarcoptes* mites and *Notoedres* are very difficult to differentiate. Both are very small (200–400 μm) and oval. In *Sarcoptes,* the first two pairs of legs are short with long unjointed stalks containing suckers. In *Notoedres,* the stalks are of medium length, and the caudal legs have long bristles. The anus is terminal in *Sarcoptes*, while it is dorsal in *Notoedres. Cheyletiella* mites are large and have four pairs of legs with combs instead of claws. The most diagnostic feature of the mite is the accessory mouthpart or palpi that terminates in hooks.

70 i. This patient is not a candidate for an intradermal skin test. According to the history, the patient is only pruritic when it has bacterial pyoderma and/or when its seborrhea is untreated. A combination of bacteria, yeast, and inflammatory by-products of oily seborrhea are causing the pruritus. An underlying nonpruritic disease causing the recurrent bacterial pyoderma, seborrhea, and hair loss should be pursued before an allergy evaluation.

ii. This is a true case. These breeders were unintentionally selecting and breeding a line of hypothyroid dachshunds. These dogs all developed recurrent bacterial and yeast infections, secondary seborrhea, and inflammatory skin changes (**70b**). Once this dog's hypothyroidism was treated, along with the secondary skin infections and seborrhea, the dog's skin was normal. He was also markedly more active and mischievous.

iii. One of the most common causes of canine hypothyroidism is lymphocytic thyroiditis, which is hereditary. These dogs should not be used for breeding, and the breeding stock in this kennel should be screened for hypothyroidism. Evaluation of antithyroglobulin antibodies, fT4, and canine TSH will be most helpful in the screening process.

71 A cat is presented for the complaint of a well-circumscribed, noninflammatory area of alopecia (71). The owner reports the hair loss waxes and wanes, and that the cat is not pruritic. Previous skin scrapings and fungal cultures have been negative. Skin biopsy findings report a predominance of catagen and telogen hair follicles, follicular atrophy, and rare peribulbar accumulations of lymphocytes, histiocytes, and plasma cells.

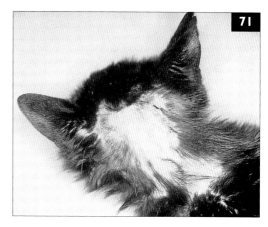

i. What are the differential diagnoses for this lesion in the cat and, based upon the skin biopsy findings, what is the most likely diagnosis?
ii. How is this disease managed?
iii. What is pseudopelade?

72 A 4-year-old cat is presented for a swollen chin. The owner reports that the cat rubs its chin on furniture, walls, and on her (72). On physical examination there is hair loss, erythema, broken whiskers, and evidence of self-trauma at the commissures of the mouth. Dermatological examination is otherwise normal. Flea combing is negative.

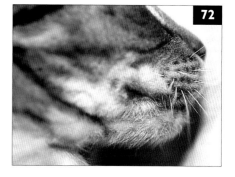

i. This cat's dermatological problem is 'facial pruritus'. What are the most common differential diagnoses? What diagnostic tests are indicated at this first visit?
ii. How should this cat be managed?

71 i. Differential diagnoses include alopecia areata, follicular dysplasia, and pseudo-pelade. If there had been a history of topical glucocorticoid use, then a localized steroid endocrinopathy could be included in the differential diagnosis. If the lesion shown was in an area where the cat could groom, psychogenic alopecia/overgrooming would also be a reasonable differential diagnosis. The histological findings are most compatible with alopecia areata. Skin biopsy findings usually include a description of a predominance of catagen and telogen hair follicles, follicular atrophy, and rare peribulbar accumulations of lymphocytes, histiocytes, and plasma cells.

ii. Alopecia areata is believed to be an immune-mediated disease that targets follicular antigens, causing destruction of the hair follicles. These lesions tend to wax and wane and may regrow hair spontaneously. There is no effective therapy.

iii. Pseudopelade is an immune-mediated disease of dogs and cats that is characterized by well-circumscribed noninflammatory alopecia (dogs) and symmetrical alopecia (cats). Immunological studies show there are high numbers of $\alpha\beta$, CD8+ lymphocytes within the epithelium of the hair follicle as well as CD1+ dendritic cells. In addition, circulating IgG antibodies against keratin and trichohylanin have been reported (Power et al., 1998; Gross et al., 2000).

72 i. The differential diagnoses include: food allergy, atopy, demodicosis, bacterial pyoderma, *Malassezia* dermatitis, dermatophytosis, dental or gingival disease, and mastocytoma or 'fat chin disease'. FAD is not a likely cause. In cats, FAD can be localized to the head and neck, but the author is unaware of any cases that involve localization to only the chin. *Notoedres* mites can cause facial pruritus, but usually there is more extensive involvement of the head and crusting of the skin often occurs. Skin scraping for *Demodex* mites, impression smears for bacteria and/or yeast, a dermatophyte culture, and a thorough oral examination for dental or gingival disease should all be done in cats with facial pruritus.

ii. The first thing to determine is whether or not the excessive chin rubbing is caused by a nondermatological problem such as gingivitis or dental disease. If dental disease is ruled out, treatment of any secondary bacterial or yeast infection found on cytological smears is the next course of action. There are large concentrations of sebaceous glands in the face and chin and colonization with bacteria and yeast is common. These infections can be very pruritic, and it is important to eliminate secondary causes of pruritus before pursuing more advanced diagnostic testing. A skin biopsy may rule out less likely causes of pruritus, such as mastocytosis. Assuming there is no infection, or if the cat is still pruritic after treatment of the infections, the cat should be evaluated for atopy and/or a food allergy. This was a case of feline atopy. This cat was found to be allergic to house dust. It responded to immunotherapy for house dust/house dust mites.

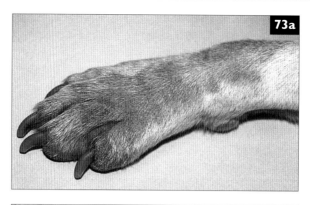

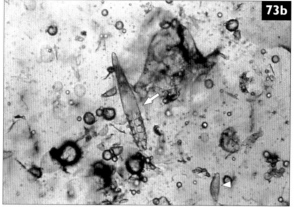

73 The foreleg of a 16-week-old puppy presented because of nonpruritic hair loss is shown (73a). A mite was found on skin scraping (73b, arrow). Skin scrapings of other areas of the body were negative for mites.
i. What is the diagnosis?
ii. What are the treatment options?
iii. The mechanism of action of amitraz makes contact with this drug dangerous for people taking certain medications. What is the mechanism of action of this drug, what are the common adverse effects, and what is the antidote for overdose?

74 There are two major categories of adverse drug reactions. What are they? Give an example of each type.

73 i. Localized demodicosis. This diagnosis was based upon the fact that lesions are few in number, and mites are localized to only the affected area. An adult *Demodex* mite can be seen along with a lemon-shaped egg (**73b**, arrowhead).

ii. The best course of treatment is difficult to determine in cases of localized demodicosis. Conservative treatment would involve a 'watch and wait' approach. This appears to be a case of localized demodicosis because there is only one lesion present and mites were not found in normal adjacent skin. Approximately 90% of cases will self-cure without treatment. If this puppy were otherwise healthy, this would be an appropriate treatment approach. If more lesions develop, a more aggressive treatment approach can be used.

Aggressive therapy would involve treating the puppy with weekly amitraz dips until there are at least three negative skin scrapings at weekly intervals. Although there are numerous treatments for demodicosis, weekly amitraz dips are still the best initial approach. Alternative therapies (ivermectin, milbemycin) should be reserved for patients that do not respond to amitraz therapy. The author does not consider alternative therapies until patients have received at least 5 months of therapy (20 dips) and live mites and/or multiple life stages are present. Other considerations for using alternative therapy would include whether or not the dog is tractable to be treated topically or if the owner can afford topical therapy. Amitraz should be applied by a veterinarian or a technician directly under the supervision of a veterinarian. Although this appears to be a localized lesion, it is rather large and immature mites (e.g. eggs) were found on the skin scraping. It could be argued that starting therapy at this time would be prudent to prevent or minimize the chance that this animal goes on to develop generalized demodicosis.

iii. Amitraz is a monoamine oxidase inhibitor. It inhibits prostaglandin synthesis, and it is an alpha-adrenergic agonist. This drug also inhibits insulin release, explaining why dogs experience transient polyuria and polydipsia. Other adverse effects include sedation, pruritus, urticaria, weakness, ataxia, and bradycardia. People taking monoamine oxidase inhibitors or who have glucose regulation disorders should not come into contact with this drug. Yohimbine and atipamezole, along with supportive care, are used in cases of overdose or to treat dogs with severe adverse effects.

74 Adverse drug reactions can be divided into predictable and unpredictable/idiosyncratic reactions. Predictable adverse drug reactions are usually dose related and are often related to the pharmacology of the drug. An example would be the vomiting associated with xylazine hydrochloride. Unpredictable or idiosyncratic drug reactions are dose independent and are related to the host's immune response and/or the breed of the dog. An example would be ivermectin sensitivity in collie dogs.

75 A 10-year-old female spayed poodle dog is brought in for a 'wart vaccine' appointment after 'catching warts after grooming'. Further questioning of the client reveals the dog has no history of having viral papillomatosis as a puppy. The current lesions have been slowly developing as the dog has aged. The lesions are most obvious to the owner after the dog's hair coat has been trimmed, and also because they are traumatized during grooming. The dog's

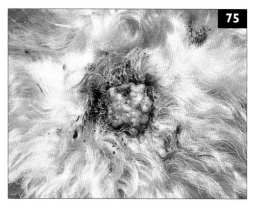

hair coat is slightly oily. The owner is repeatedly requesting the 'wart vaccine'. Close examination of the skin reveals multiple, well-circumscribed, raised, cauliflower-like lesions (75). The lesions are freely movable in the dermis, and the dog has approximately 15 such lesions.

i. What is this lesion, what should be the response to the owner's request for a 'wart vaccine', and what is the prognosis?

ii. What are the four syndromes in dogs that are associated with viral papillomatosis?

iii. Autogenous papilloma vaccines have been used to treat true cases of oral papillomatosis. What is the risk associated with the use of these vaccines?

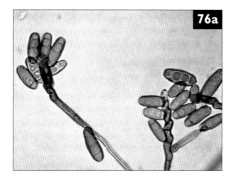

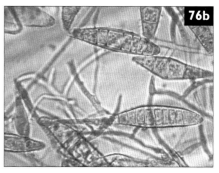

76 Microscopic views of two fungal organisms are shown (76a, b).

i. Based on the colony morphology presented, which one of these organisms is a contaminant and which one is a pathogen. Why?

ii. How was this preparation made?

75 i. This is an example of nodular sebaceous gland hyperplasia. This is the second most common skin tumor in dogs. It is common in breeds such as beagles, cocker spaniels, poodles, dachshunds, and miniature schnauzers. The cause is unknown, but lesions are common in older dogs and dogs with seborrheic skin disease. Diagnosis can be confirmed by finding clusters of lipidized sebocytes on FNA or by excisional biopsy. These are not warts, and there is no 'vaccine' for these lesions. Such lesions are best left untreated or, if traumatized, removed surgically. The prognosis is good since sebaceous gland hyperplasia is a benign skin lesion. Lesions can be observed and not treated, or removed surgically (using blade, laser, electrosurgery). Although new lesions may develop, tumors do not recur at the site of removal.
ii. 'Warts' in dogs are caused by a papillomavirus. There are four syndromes recognized in dogs: oral lesions in puppies that self-cure, horn-like lesions on the footpads of dogs 1–2 years of age, pigmented papules, plaques or nodules on the body of dogs 3–5 years of age, and an ocular form that occurs in dogs of any age, but usually in younger to middle-aged dogs. Immunotherapy (papillomavirus vaccine) has not been effective for treatment or prevention of these viral lesions.
iii. The efficacy of autogenous vaccines has always been in question because the lesions, at least in puppies, spontaneously regress. The risk associated with the use of these vaccines stems from the finding of neoplasms (squamous papilloma, basal cell epithelioma, and squamous cell carcinoma) at the site of injection of the live vaccine (Bregman *et al.*, 1987).

76 i. The heavily pigmented organism is not a dermatophyte, it is a fungal contaminant (76a). Fungal contaminants can be darkly pigmented, pale, or vary in color from green to blue to yellow depending upon the species. Dermatophytes are never grossly or microscopically darkly pigmented. The pale blue organism is a macro conidia of *Microsporum canis* (76b). Note the 'boat' shaped appearance of the macro conidia. *M. canis* typically has six or more cells, tapered ends, and thick walls. In contrast, *M. gypseum* has less than six cells and is thin walled. These differentiating characteristics may be hard to see in young colony growth. Because some fungal contaminants, such as *Aspergillus* spp. mimic fungal pathogens, microscopic identification of suspect pathogens using lactophenol cotton blue should always be done.
ii. Microscopic identification of fungal organisms is easily performed in practice. Clear acetate tape is gently pressed against the colony growth and then placed on a glass microscope slide over a drop of lactophenol cotton blue stain. This stain is called a vital stain because it is used on living organisms; the phenol kills the fungal spores on contact. Care must be taken when using this stain, as it will damage a microscope lens.

77 A close-up view of the skin of a dog presented for a second opinion is shown (77). The dog has a 1 year history of generalized pruritus and seborrhea. Previous skin scrapings have been negative. The pruritus and seborrhea were treated with glucocorticoids and antiseborrhea shampoos, but the lesions persisted and/or returned shortly after discontinuation of therapy. Examination of the medical records

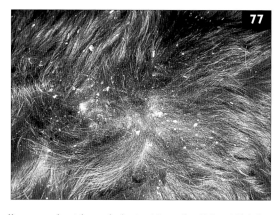

reveals that the dog was repeatedly treated with cephalexin (5 mg/kg PO q12h) for 7–10 days. Close examination of the skin reveals easily epilated hairs, scattered papules, hairs piercing the scales, and a mild odor.
i. Given the information provided, what is the most likely cause of this patient's recurrent seborrhea and pruritus, and what diagnostics should be performed to confirm the diagnosis?
ii. What information in the history may explain why the infection is recurrent? How should this skin disease be treated?
iii. Why is topical therapy beneficial in the treatment of bacterial pyoderma, and what treatment options are available for this patient?

78 The forepaws of an adult cat are shown (78).
i. What is this condition called?
ii. What treatment, if any, is required?

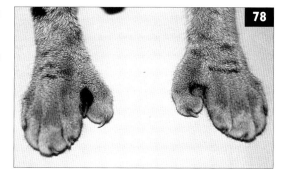

77 i. Superficial bacterial pyoderma. Hair piercing scales are a common finding in animals with pustular skin diseases, the most common of which is a bacterial infection. Skin scrapings should be repeated in this patient to rule out demodicosis as an underlying cause, or as the result of the chronic steroid therapy. Flea combings should be performed to look for *Cheyletiella* mites, fleas, and lice as either underlying causes of the pyoderma or complicating secondary skin disease. Impression smears should be done to rule out a concurrent yeast infection.

ii. The most commonly encountered errors in the treatment of bacterial pyoderma include: concurrent use of glucocorticoids with antibiotic therapy, using too low a dose of antibiotics, too short a course of antibiotic therapy, and an ineffective drug. All but the latter occurred in this case. Other important causes of treatment failure include lack of pursuit of an underlying disease, concurrent *Malassezia* dermatitis that was not diagnosed and/or treated, and misdiagnosis of pyoderma.

This patient's pruritus and seborrhea were 'cured' with a 6 week treatment course of oral antibiotics, topical antibacterial shampoo therapy (alternate chlorhexidine and benzoyl peroxide shampoo), and immediate discontinuation of the glucocorticoids. Yeast organisms were not found on impression smears.

iii. Topical shampoo therapy removes debris and crusts from the epidermis. These can be heavily laden with bacteria. It removes bacteria from the surface of the skin, follicular infundibula, and helps remove debris from deep draining tracts. Shampoo therapy has a soothing effect on pruritic skin, especially when applied with tepid water. The author instructs clients to pre-dilute the shampoo before applying to the patient. This minimizes the potential for shampoo residue on the hair coat and the development of irritant reactions from the application of concentrated shampoo to inflamed skin. Benzoyl peroxide, ethyl lactate, chlorhexidine, sulfur, and salicylic acid are the main ingredients in antibacterial shampoos.

78 i. Polydactyly. This is a hereditary disorder seen in cats in which there is an extra digit. Affected cats appear to have 'thumbs'. A common lay term for this condition is 'mittened'.

ii. This condition is cosmetic and causes the cat no discomfort provided that the claws of the extra toes do not grow into the associated pad. Owners should be educated that they need to look at the cat's claws and cut the nails, as needed. If the nail does grow into the pad, the cat will become lame. This is easily solved by a nail trim, but in severe cases, the cat may be in pain and require sedation or a short-acting anesthetic. Owners are very fond of the appearance of these cats, and although surgical removal of the extra digit will prevent in-grown claws, owners often prefer not to have this done.

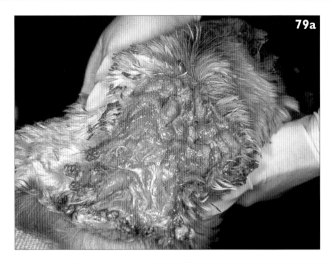

79 The inner pinna of a 10-year-old cocker spaniel dog is shown; both ears are similar in appearance (79a). The owners report the dog has a history of ear infections, and they noticed the proliferation starting on the inner pinnae about 3 years ago. The ears are exudative, malodorous, and the ear canal feels calcified upon palpation. The dog is experiencing a great deal of pain. Calcification of the soft tissue of the ear is confirmed on skull radiographs (79b, arrows).

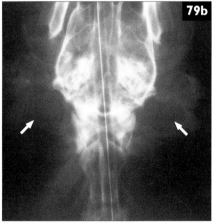

i. What type of ear disease is represented here?
ii. What are the treatment options?

80 Insect growth regulators and insect development inhibitors are used in flea control.
i. What is the difference between an insect growth regulator and insect development inhibitor?
ii. Give examples of each class of drugs.
iii. What are the advantages and disadvantages of each class of drugs?

79 i. This is a case of severe proliferative otitis. The severity of the proliferation and calcification of the ear canal is compatible with what is called 'end stage ear disease'. It is highly probable there is a mixed bacterial infection complicating the situation. Otitis media is highly likely in this patient.

ii. The treatment options in this patient are very limited. In patients with end stage ear disease, TECA and BO are recommended. In this patient, there is marked proliferation and calcification of the lining of the ear canal and the lining of the inner pinnae. TECA and BO along with surgical amputation of the ear pinnae were recommended to the client as the only viable treatment option. In this case, the clients elected euthanasia.

80 i. Insect growth regulators are analogues of the insect juvenile hormone. In the normal development of a flea, a fall in juvenile hormone concentrations triggers the development of the pupal stage. These drugs prevent pupation and they are also ovicidal. Insect development inhibitors affect nonadult stages of the life cycle by means other than affecting pupation.

ii. The most commonly used insect growth regulators are fenoxycarb, methoprene, and pyriproxifen. Methoprene and pyriproxifen can be used on animals and are available in collars or topical products. Fenoxycarb is used in the environment. The most commonly known insect development inhibitors are lufenuron and cyromazine. Lufenuron is a benzylphenol that inhibits chitin, an important component of the flea exoskeleton. Cyromazine is an aminotriazine. It does not inhibit chitin but rather causes the exoskeleton to become stiff and results in lethal body wall defects. It is not widely used.

iii. Methoprene is directly and indirectly ovidial, embryocidal, and larvicidal. It does not readily wash off the animal or surfaces to which it has been applied. The product is safe for use on cats and can be used in combination with other products. The major disadvantages of the drug include sensitivity to ultraviolet radiation and that it can volatilize and move to other locations. Pyriproxyfen is ovicidal and larvicidal and is not sensitive to ultraviolet radiation. It is very stable even outdoors and is also safe for use on cats. It is not easily removed by bathing and will translocate to bedding. The major concern about this drug is its potential to harm nontarget species insects.

Insect growth regulators are systemic drugs that have high margins of safety. They are an alternative to environmental insecticides although it can take greater than 3 months for fleas to be eliminated from a closed home environment. There is no residue problem on animals or people and they are safe for use in cats. The major disadvantage of this drug is that it must be given with food to be absorbed, takes months to eliminate fleas from the environment, it has no adulticidal activity, and animals can bring new fleas into the home (Kunkle and Halliwell, 2002).

81 The owners of a 3-year-old spayed female dachshund dog presented her for the problem of symmetrical nonpruritic hair loss (81a). Upon examination, the skin was thin, the dog was slightly 'pot bellied', and the superficial vasculature on the ventral abdomen was more prominent than expected (81b, c). The dog sunbathes, and the owner reported no changes in the dog's water consumption, urination, defecation, or behavior. A complete blood count, urinalysis, and serum chemistry panel were ordered, and all values were within normal limits. The skin biopsy finding was 'compatible with an endocrine alopecia'. The epidermis and dermis were thin, and the hair follicles were atrophied.

i. What are the differential diagnoses for nonpruritic symmetrical alopecia in this breed?

ii. Why were the screening diagnostic tests ordered for this patient? Additional diagnostic testing is indicated in this patient. What tests should be ordered?

iii. What is a UCCR, and how might the information be useful in treating this patient?

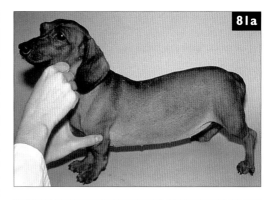

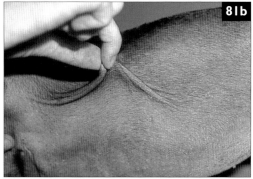

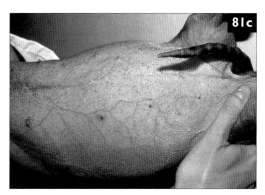

81: Answer

81 i. The differential diagnoses include hypothyroidism, hyperadrenocorticism, pattern alopecia, and estrogen-responsive alopecia. Hyperadrenocorticism and hypothyroidism are the two most common endocrine disorders in this breed, and in the early stages they can look very similar. Pattern alopecia is a hereditary disorder common in this breed. It usually presents with bilaterally symmetrical hair loss over the head, ears, ventrum, and caudal thigh. Estrogen-responsive dermatosis is very rare, but it has been reported in this breed also. It would be a diagnosis of elimination.

ii. The most likely cause of this patient's hair loss is an endocrine disorder; however, the history and clinical signs do not allow differentiation between canine hypothyroidism and hyperadrenocorticism. The dog's clinical signs are very suggestive of hyperadrenocorticism, but the dog is rather young for this problem and is not showing any other symptoms except for hair loss, thin skin, and a slight pot-bellied appearance. The history of sunbathing suggests hypothyroidism. However, the heat seeking behavior could be due to the fact the dog is simply cold because it has lost its hair due to a nonendocrine follicular disorder.

A complete blood count, urinalysis, serum chemistry panel, and skin biopsy are indicated to help differentiate causes of endocrine hair loss from follicular diseases. A thyroid screening panel, low-dose dexamethasone test, and an ACTH stimulation test would be the next series of tests. A thyroid screening panel was ordered first in this patient and was found to be normal. An ACTH stimulation test was performed next and was normal. The results of the low-dose dexamethasone suppression test (0.01 mg/kg IV) revealed an elevated basal cortisol at 0 hours, marked suppression of cortisol at 4 hours post-dexamethasone, and an elevated cortisol concentration at 8 hours post-dexamethasone. These findings not only answer the question of whether or not the dog has hyperadrenocorticism but also were compatible with PDH. In a normal dog, the 8 hour cortisol concentration would be suppressed, but in this case, it was not. A high-dose dexamethasone suppression test (0.1 mg/kg IV) confirmed this was a case of PDH. (The high-dose dexamethasone suppression test in this patient was optional as the low-dose dexamethasone suppression test was compatible with PDH.)

iii. A UCCR is a screening test that rules out hyperadrenocorticism. Dogs with spontaneous hyperadrenocorticism have an elevated UCCR, but most dogs with an elevated UCCR do not have hyperadrenocorticism. If the test is normal, it is most likely the dog does not have hyperadrenocorticism. If the test is elevated, adrenal function tests are indicated to answer the question of whether or not the dog has hyperadrenocorticism. An abnormal UCCR test would have signaled that adrenal function testing is needed, saving the owner the cost of the skin biopsy and thyroid function testing.

82 A 2-year-old cocker spaniel
dog was presented for the complaint of bilateral epiphora and
periocular pruritus (82). On
physical examination, mild signs
of primary seborrhea were noted
(nasal digital hyperkeratosis and
scaling). The discharge in the
periocular area was thick and
malodorous, and impression
smears of this area revealed bacterial and yeast organisms. The
initial working diagnosis was

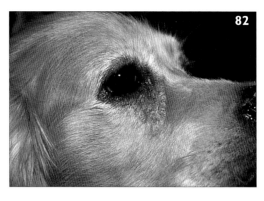

primary seborrhea with mild facial fold pyoderma. The epiphora and periocular
pruritus did not resolve after a 21 day course of oral antibiotics and ketoconazole;
however, impression smears of the skin revealed that the microbial infection had
resolved. Closer examination of the patient revealed there was no evidence of face
rubbing, chewing, or whole body pruritus. The dog's conjunctivae were reddened,
and the sclera injected. Excessive tearing was noted. What are two common causes of
epiphora in this breed of dog?

83 A 4-year-old male mixed
breed dog is presented as an
emergency with a skin lesion on
its lateral left thigh. The owners
left for dinner 4 hours ago, and
when they returned, the dog was
biting and chewing at this lesion.
The dog is extremely agitated
with a 10 × 7 cm lesion on its
lateral left thigh. The lesion is
extremely painful, pruritic, and
exudative (83).
i. What is the clinical diagnosis?
ii. How should this lesion be
treated?

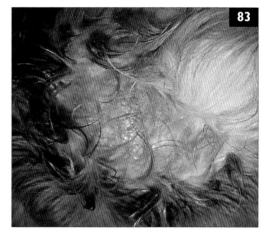

82 The two most common causes of epiphora in this breed are blockage of the nasal lacrimal duct and distichiasis. This dog's nasal lacrimal duct was patent. Careful examination of the patient under mild sedation revealed severe distichia on both the lower and upper eyelid. This case of distichiasis was treated by electroepilation of the cilia.

83 i. The lesion is most compatible with an area of pyotruamatic dermatitis (hot spot). There are two 'classifications' of pyotraumatic dermatitis in veterinary dermatology: pyotraumatic dermatitis and pyotraumatic folliculitis. Pyotraumatic dermatitis is described clinically as an acute, flat, ulcerative lesion with surface colonization of bacteria but not follicular invasion. In the case of pyotraumatic folliculitis, the lesions can look similar, but satellite lesions of folliculitis are present, and bacteria have invaded the hair follicles. It is the author's opinion that the classification is academic as an untreated or inappropriately treated lesion of pyotraumatic dermatitis will develop into an area of pyotraumatic folliculitis and furunculosis, i.e. one lesion is simply the early form of the other.

ii. Pyotraumatic lesions develop acutely and are very pruritic and painful. The dog should be sedated and the hair from the area clipped. The lesion should be washed with a mild antibacterial scrub and topical antibiotic ointment applied. Topical drying agents (astringents) delay epithelial migration and slow healing of the wound, so their use should be avoided. Cleaning of the wound is a key step in breaking the infamous 'itch-scratch' cycle. Many dogs will no longer traumatize these areas after they have been cleaned. The wound should be covered with a protective ointment or dressing. The application of a topical antibiotic ointment (e.g. mupiricin) is preferred because it does not inhibit epithelial migration. Also, these ointments act as wound barriers and cover the free nerve endings in the epidermis; much of the pain and pruritus in these lesions is due to the exposure of free nerve endings. Some clinicians prefer to use a glucocorticoid containing product. Finally, the decision about use of systemic antibiotic therapy needs to be made. Not all clinicians feel that systemic antibiotic therapy is needed in the treatment of acute focal pyotraumatic dermatitis. It is the author's preference always to treat these lesions as areas of pyoderma, as a careful and thorough dermatological examination almost always reveals evidence of concurrent bacterial pyoderma, underlying pruritic disease, or evidence of satellite lesions of folliculitis as a result of the traumatic lesions. In long and/or heavy coated dogs, pyotraumatic lesions are areas of deep pyoderma, and systemic antibiotic therapy for 4 weeks or more is the treatment of choice. The use of concurrent glucocorticoids in the treatment of bacterial pyoderma is contraindicated; however, in this condition it may be necessary to administer oral glucocorticoids for 24–48 hours in some patients to provide humane relief of pain and pruritus. This is especially true in situations where lesions develop in a matter of hours. (See also 84.)

84 With regard to the case of pyotraumatic dermatitis in 83:
i. Recurrent lesions of this type are commonly seen in what disease(s)?
ii. What two diseases can present as areas of chronic recurrent pyotraumatic derma-titis and are diagnosed via skin biopsy?

85 A 9-month-old cat is presented for the lesion seen on its face (85). The owner reports that the lesion developed over the last 24 hours. The owner also reports the cat has had similar facial lesions previously, but never one this severe or acute. This is an indoor cat, and the only other pet in the house is a canary. The owner practices flea control even though the cat does not go outside. The only change in the cat's environment and husbandry was a diet change from a nonpre-scription over the counter canned cat food to a prescription lamb-

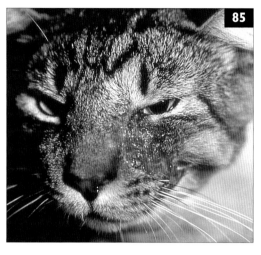

and chicken-based dry cat food. The lesion is pruritic, and blood and hair are trapped in the cat's hind claws. Physical examination is otherwise normal. Skin scrapings and flea combings are negative. Impression smears revealed septic inflammation with intracellular cocci. A dermatophyte culture is pending. The initial working diagnosis is bacterial pyoderma, and the cat is treated with liquid cephalexin (30 mg/kg PO q12h) for 21 days. The lesion resolves, but the cat is still pruritic and within 10 days of completing the antibiotic therapy, another lesion develops. Bacterial cultures of the lesion are negative. Impression smears reveal neutrophilic and eosinophilic inflam-mation but no visible organisms. Fungal culture results are negative.
i. What is/are this cat's dermatological problem(s)?
ii. What differential diagnoses can be eliminated at this point?
iii. What else should be examined prior to pursuing additional dermatological testing? Assuming no other physical abnormalities are found, what diagnostic tests should be performed?

84 i. The most common causes of recurrent areas of pyotraumatic dermatitis are inappropriate therapy for the original lesions, unresolved bacterial pyoderma and/or an unrecognized pruritic disease such as atopy, food allergy, and/or fleas. Recurrent facial 'hotspots' due to atopy are common in thick coated breeds such as golden retrievers, Labrador retrievers, and Newfoundland dogs.

ii. Areas of resolving calcinosis cutis and apocrine gland carcinomas can present as nonhealing areas of pyotraumatic dermatitis/folliculitis.

85 i. Facial pruritus.

ii. Skin scrapings, flea combings, and monthly flea control eliminate demodicosis, flea infestation, *Cheyletiella*, stick tight fleas, and lice as underlying causes. *Otodectes* infestation of the ears is still possible, although unlikely in an indoor cat receiving monthly flea control and without exposure to other cats. The negative fungal culture rules out dermatophytosis; *Microsporum canis* can cause eosinophilic plaque-like lesions. The fact that the cat was still pruritic after antibiotic therapy resolved the acute septic lesion indicates there is an underlying pruritic trigger for these lesions. The use of flea control makes FAD unlikely.

iii. Under anesthesia, the cat's external and middle ear canal should be examined. Some cats with intense facial pruritus have eosinophilic plaques in the ear canal. Ears should be examined for foreign bodies or tumors that will cause the cat to traumatize itself. In addition, cats with undiagnosed *Malassezia* otitis or ear mites can develop lesions on the face. The cat's eyes should be carefully examined for any abnormalities, particularly distichiasis.

Several options exist for further diagnostic testing. If the clinician and/or owner are still unsure about the origin of the lesion, unstained impression smears and a skin biopsy could be submitted to a diagnostic laboratory for confirmation. (In this case, the owner requested that the lesion be confirmed; it was an eosinophilic plaque). In this patient, both food allergy and/or atopy could be the cause of the recurrent facial lesions. Because of the young age of the cat, and because at least one of the episodes was triggered by a diet change, a restricted diet trial was recommended. This cat's eosinophilic plaque was treated with an injection of methylprednisone acetate (20 mg/cat SC) followed by a 10 week diet trial using a canned rabbit diet. At the end of the trial, the cat was normal and no further lesions developed. The cat was challenged with its previous diet, and within 72 hours, it began furiously scratching at its face creating another eosinophilic plaque. This cat was diagnosed with a food allergy. The owner was not interested in identifying the specific offending food and elected to continue feeding the canned rabbit diet.

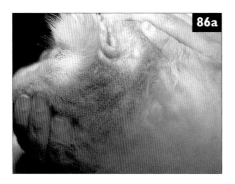
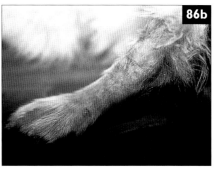

86 A 10-week-old chow chow puppy is presented for hair loss, erythema, itching behind the right ear (**86a**), and on the right rear foot (**86b**). An area of ulceration on the digit is also present, and the owner reported the wound was self-inflicted. Upon questioning, the owner reports that the lesions slowly developed over 2 weeks, and that hair loss preceded pruritus.

i. What are the differential diagnoses, and what diagnostic tests are indicated?

ii. Closer examination of the skin revealed that follicular plugging caused hyperpigmentation in this patient. What skin diseases are associated with follicular plugging?

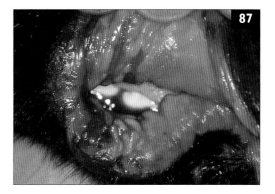

87 A German shepherd dog was presented for examination because of mouth odor and drooling. Upon dermatological examination, the skin was odorous, exudative, and erosions on the mucocutaneous margins (mouth, eyelids, and anus) were present (**87**). The dog was otherwise healthy.

i. What is the diagnosis and how should this problem be treated?

ii. What dog breeds may be at greater risk for developing mucocutaneous pyoderma?

iii. How is this bacterial disease different from lip fold pyoderma? How would a biopsy specimen differentiate lip fold pyoderma from mucocutaneous pyoderma?

86 i. This puppy has two major dermatological problems: pruritus and hair loss. The most common causes of hair loss in puppies are demodicosis, dermatophytosis, and bacterial pyoderma. The most common causes of pruritus include flea infestation, demodicosis, scabies, cheyletiellosis, dermatophytosis, and bacterial pyoderma.

The diagnostics tests indicated are deep skin scrapings for demodicosis, impressions smears to look for yeast and/or cocci, and a dermatophyte culture. This is a case of dermatophytosis due to *Microsporum gypseum*. The puppy contracted this dermatophyte while at the breeder's home since several other littermates and the bitch also developed lesions. The puppies were also housed outside in a pen with a dirt floor. *M. gypseum* is a geophilic organism, and animals contract it from exposure to contaminated soil, often through digging. This puppy was treated successfully with topical lime sulfur dips twice a week, for 8 weeks. The puppy was treated until two negative fungal cultures were obtained at 2 week intervals. Systemic antifungal therapy was not used in this puppy because it was <12 weeks of age. It is also important to inform the owner that this is a zoonotic disease.

ii. Follicular plugging with black debris is common in demodicosis, *Malassezia* dermatitis, bacterial pyoderma, and seborrheic skin diseases.

87 i. Mucocutaneous pyoderma. This presentation tends to start on the lips, but may also occur on any mucocutaneous area (vulva, eyelids, nares, prepuce, or anus). The tissue is swollen, exudative, and painful. Concurrent infections with *Staphylococcus intermedius* and *Malassezia* are common. It is important to consider other differential diagnoses such as lupus erythematosus, lip fold pyoderma, zinc responsive dermatoses, early PF, drug reactions, candidiasis, and erythema multiforme. Diagnosis is confirmed by response to antimicrobial therapy and, if necessary, skin biopsy. Severe cases can be very painful and may mimic more life-threatening diseases. Differentiation from lip fold pyoderma may be difficult, but the lack of chronicity and anatomical folds may be helpful. Systemic antibiotics for at least 4 weeks are indicated. Concurrent topical therapy with mupirocin ointment and antibacterial soaks may be helpful.

ii. This can occur in any breed of dog, but German shepherd dogs and German shepherd dog crosses appear to be predisposed.

iii. Lip fold pyoderma is caused by anatomical apposition of tissues, and lesions are localized to areas where the redundant skin causes friction. There is usually a history of chronicity. In lip fold pyoderma, lesions are, by definition, localized to the lip fold area. Concurrent involvement of other mucocutaneous junctions eliminates this as a differential diagnosis. In mucocutaneous pyoderma, there is dense plasmactyic, lichenoid dermatitis in the dermis that is not present in the dermis of a lip fold pyoderma.

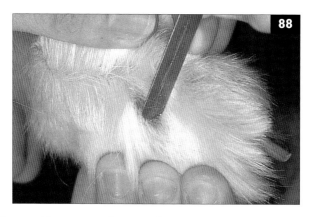

88 What is the metal instrument shown in the picture (88)?

89 Mucocutaneous ulcerations, either focal or multifocal, are a major dermatological problem (89a, b).
i. What are the major differential diagnoses for mucocutaneous ulceration in either the dog or cat?
ii. What other dermatological diagnostic tests, other than skin biopsy, should be done when evaluating a patient with mucocutaneous ulcerations?
iii. What is epidermolysis bullosa acquista?

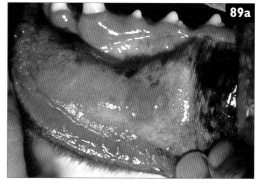

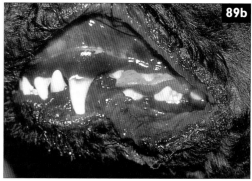

88, 89: Answers

88 The flat metal instrument is a skin-scraping spatula. This can be purchased from medical or chemical suppliers, and it is also used as a weighing spatula. This tool is used for obtaining superficial and deep skin scrapings. There are a number of advantages of the metal spatula over a traditional scalpel blade. First, the spatula is reusable and less expensive than using a new scalpel blade for every patient. Second, and more importantly, it is safer method for collecting specimens for both the patient and clinician. The edge of the blade is sharp enough for scraping the skin, but not sharp enough to cut either the patient or clinician. This tool is especially useful in small or struggling patients that may be easily injured. Another use of the tool is for the collection of cytological specimens from beneath nail beds, crevices in the skin, or for collection of surface material. It also is extremely difficult to obtain safely a sample of nail bed debris or exudate from interdigital areas or fold and crevices in the skin with a scalpel blade.

89 i. In cases of oral mucocutaneous ulceration, the most important differential diagnosis to rule out first is oral ulceration due to renal failure. The immunological diseases associated with mucocutaneous ulceration include pemphigus vulgaris, bullous pemphigoid, systemic lupus erythematosus, and erythema multiforme. Drug eruptions, heptocutaneous syndrome, thallium toxicity, and cutaneous lymphoma can also cause local or generalized mucocutaneous ulcerations. Several diseases caused by infectious agents must also be considered, including leishmaniasis, prototheccosis, phaeohyphomycosis, staphylococcal infection, and candidiasis.
ii. As mentioned above, serum chemistries to rule out renal failure should be done in any case involving oral ulceration. Second, cytological preparations of exudates from the margins of lesions should be examined for the presence of cocci, *Malassezia*, and/or *Candida*. These preparations are made by gently scraping the edge of a lesion, smearing the exudate on a glass microscope slide and staining after air-drying. Candidiasis may need to be confirmed via fungal culture. Mucocutaneous candidiasis is often associated with an underlying systemic disease, e.g. neoplasia, immune-mediated disease, or immunosuppression.
iii. Mucuous membrane pemphigoid is increasingly being recognized as a major immune-mediated disease of dogs and cats. It causes mucous membrane ulceration comprised of vesicles, erosions, and ulcers that are present around the oral cavity, eyes, ears, anus, and genitalia. Most animals are affected by 1 year of age and German shepherd dogs are predisposed. Histologically, the disease is characterized by subepidermal vesiculation. Immunological tests to confirm the disease include finding basement membrane bound IgG via direct or immunoperoxidase testing methods.

90 It is late spring, and the local television stations have been televising public service announcements about the dangers of sunbathing. The television commercials included a list of various types of skin tumors that can develop in people as a result of excessive sun exposure (e.g. basal cell tumors, squamous cell carcinomas, melanoma). People with any suspicious lesions are urged to seek a consultation with their physician. One day, a very distressed owner calls and requests a 'skin cancer check' for her dog. During the examination, she points out a raised, solitary, pigmented lesion that has rapidly developed on the dorsum of her West Highland white terrier dog (90).

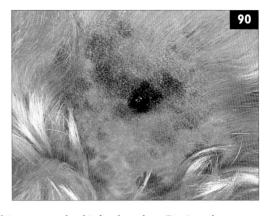

i. What is the most likely diagnosis and how should this lesion be managed?
ii. What role does breed play in predicting prognostic significance?
iii. What roles does lesion location have in predicting benign or malignant behavior?

91 An indoor-outdoor cat is presented for a facial lesion (91). The lesion is hard and adherent to the skin. However, it can be gently lifted at the margins, and a healthy granulation bed of tissue is present beneath it. There is no exudate beneath the lesion or odor present. This is the only cat in the household, there are no children in the house, and no known exposure to trauma. The only heat source in the home is a wood stove. The cat frequently sleeps as close as it can get to the wood stove.

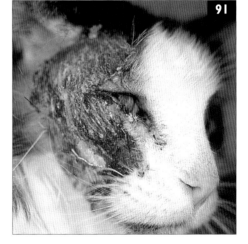

i. What is the differential diagnosis?
ii. How should the case be managed?
iii. What breed of dog has been reported recently to be at risk for ultraviolet light thermal injuries?

90 i. The most likely cause is a melanocytic neoplasm or cutaneous melanoma. Cutaneous melanomas can be benign or malignant. Benign lesions (also called melanocytoma) are usually well-defined, deeply pigmented, <2.0 cm in diameter, and mobile. Areas of pigmentation that are congenital and are most likely part of a dog's normal skin coloration are called melanocytic nevi. The treatment of choice is radical excision, and submission of the lesion and margins for histological examination. In this patient, there are multiple areas of pigmented macules that most likely are part of the dog's normal skin coloration. Because the lesion developed in this area, it may have been present for much longer than the owner reported. One of the key findings during the examination was the clearly indurated feel of the tumor. Sites of normal pigmentation or pigmentation due to inflammatory skin disease do not feel thickened or infiltrated.

ii. Breed may have an important prognostic significance as 75% of melanomas in doberman pinscher and miniature schnauzer dogs are benign while 75% of melanomas in miniature poodle dogs are malignant (Bolon *et al.*, 1990).

iii. Over 85% of melanomas in dogs arise from the haired skin and are benign. The majority of melanomas of oral or mucocutaneous origin and about 50% of melanomas from the nail bed are malignant. Melanomas with a more malignant behavior (i.e. more likely to spread to other sites and organs) usually grow rapidly, are >2.0 cm in diameter and, histologically, have a mitotic index of >3 per 10x high power field.

91 i. The differential diagnosis in this situation is difficult. The lesion is clearly 'old' because the triggering episode occurred long enough ago for the skin to die and become hard and dry. The lesion looks like a burn eschar, but the whiskers on the cat's face are not curled, as would be expected if it were exposed to a strong heat source. It is possible that this is a thermal burn caused by the cat sleeping next to the wood stove.

ii. There is no sign of infection, and a healthy bed of granulation tissue is present. Daily hydrotherapy is recommended to keep the wound clean and allow the granulation bed to continue to develop. The eschar could be allowed to slough on its own or be debrided under general anesthesia. This wound will most likely heal without complication. New hair growth may or may not occur, depending upon the depth of the injury.

iii. Dalmatian dogs are at risk for ultraviolet light thermal injuries. Recently, full thickness burns were reported in the black haired marking areas of a dalmatian puppy and adult dog as a result of exposure to direct sunlight. It has been hypothesized that dalmatians may be at risk for this type of injury because, as a breed, they are generally white and thus, may not sense the degree of developing injury and not seek shade as often as a black haired dog (Hargis and Lewis, 1999).

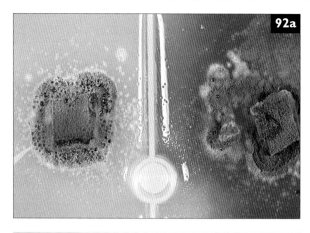

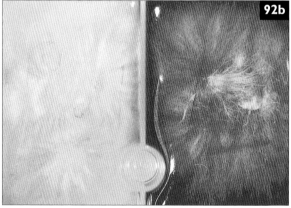

92 Two DTM plates are shown (92a, b). Both have been inoculated with a fungal culture from a dog.

i. What is DTM, and what is the principle of its use?

ii. How can the gross characteristics of fungal colony growth be used to aid in the differentiation of possible pathogens and contaminants? Which culture plate has colony growth compatible with a suspect pathogen and why?

iii. What factor may be most important in the development of false negative fungal cultures when incubated in private practice?

93 What are the clinical signs of dermatophilosis in small animals?

92 i. DTM consists of plain Sabouraud's dextrose agar, phenol red as a pH indicator, and antimicrobials to inhibit the growth of bacterial and fungal contaminants. Although there is a variety of commercially available plates, the author prefers the use of agar plates that are easy to inoculate or Sab-Duets (Bacti-Labs, Mountainview CA). The illustration shows a dual compartment plate with plain Sabouraud's dextrose agar on one side (yellow) and DTM on the other. DTM is popular because it contains a color indicator that signals the growth of a possible pathogen. Pathogens use the protein in the media first, producing the color change. In general, contaminants use the carbohydrate source first and do not produce a color change until the entire carbohydrate source has been used. The color indicator (phenol red) may alter the gross and microscopic appearance of fungal colonies and/or depress macro conidia growth. In addition, some common contaminants will grossly mimic pathogens and turn the media red.

The author avoids the use of screw top fungal culture media because they are hard to inoculate, obtain samples from, and there is an increased risk of bacterial contamination if the top is screwed on too tightly.

ii. The plate with the pale white colony is the one most compatible with a possible dermatophyte pathogen (**92b**). Dermatophyte pathogens are pale in color and are never heavily pigmented (**92a**). The red color change in the medium indicates the organism is consuming the protein in the media; both pathogens and some contaminants can turn DTM red. Contaminants tend to use the carbohydrates in the medium first before using proteins. Old fungal culture plates growing contaminants may eventually turn red as the organisms utilize the protein in the DTM.

iii. Recently a published study showed that increased incubation temperature (24–27°C [75.5–80.6°F]) resulted in a more rapid colour change on a commercial DTM developed for animals (Rapid Vet D, DMS Laboratories, Inc. Flemington, New Jersey, USA) and improved sporulation of fungi in that study (Guillot *et al.*, 2001). This study also suggested incubation at room temperature might account for false negative culture results.

93 Dermatophilosis is caused by *Dermatophilus congolensis* and is more common in horses and cattle than in dogs and cats. This disease, although rare, has been seen in warm moist climates. It is most likely to be seen in a dog or cat whose skin has been macerated and compromised by chronic wetness. Lesions are most common on the dorsum. The disease starts as erythematous papules and pustules that crust and become exudative, causing matting of the hair coat. The skin beneath these crusts is ulcerated and exudative. Diagnosis is made by finding the organism on cytological examination of skin impression smears or by culture. Treatment requires moving the host to a clean dry environment, removal of the crusts, topical antibacterial soaks, and systemic antibiotic therapy.

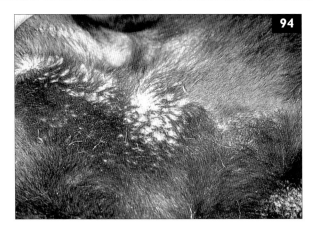

94 An adult Chinese shar-pei dog is presented for the complaint of 'blisters'. The axillary region of the dog is shown and numerous vesicles ranging in size from 0.5–>1 cm are present (94). The vesicles are firm to the touch and do not rupture easily.
i. This is a common skin condition in this breed. What is it, and how is it caused?
ii. How can it be diagnosed and managed?
iii. What causes this condition in Chinese shar-pei dogs?

95 A 2-year-old golden retriever dog is presented for the problem of acute onset of hair loss in the last 48 hours (95). The dog is nonpruritic, and the skin shows no signs of inflammation. Large amounts of hair can be pulled from the coat with normal petting. Trichogram of the shed hairs reveals they were all in the telogen phase of the hair cycle. Skin biopsy reveals large numbers of hairs in anagen. Two months

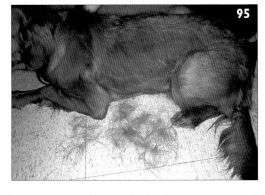

prior to presentation the dog had an intestinal foreign body that was removed surgically.
i. What is the diagnosis?
ii. How should this disorder be treated?
iii. What are the five classifications of anagen and telogen defluxion in humans?

94 i. Although this resembles an autoimmune vesicular disease, it is actually cutaneous mucinosis. Chinese shar-pei dogs have an excessive amount of dermal mucin, which gives them their characteristic 'wrinkled' appearance. The vesicles contain dermal mucin that has percolated from the dermis through the basement membrane and into the epidermis, creating a subcorneal 'vesicle'. They commonly occur in frictional areas.

ii. The easiest way to diagnose cutaneous mucinosis is to puncture gently one of the vesicles with a sterile needle and express the contents. The mucin is thick, clear, and stringy. This is a cosmetic problem and requires no treatment. In some cases, the lesions can become large and pendulous, especially when they occur on the hocks. The more wrinkled the dog, the more likely for these cosmetic lesions to be large. Oral prednisone (2 mg/kg) for 7–10 days followed by a slow reduction over 30–45 days will decrease mucin production. However, this will occur over the dog's entire body, not just in focal areas, and owners should be warned that their dogs will lose some of their wrinkled appearance. Owners often refer to this as 'deflating' their Chinese shar-pei dog.

iii. The mucinosis of Chinese shar-pei dogs is the result of massive accumulations of hyaluronic acid along with chondroitins-4 and -6 sulfate, and dermatan sulfate (Scott *et al.*, 2001f).

95 i. This is a case of telogen defluxion. This is a unique syndrome in which a severe illness, drug, high fever, shock, surgery, anesthesia, or other stressful event causes a disruption of the hair growth cycle and a sudden loss of hair several months later. The hairs abruptly stop growing, and large numbers are synchronized in catagen and then in telogen. Approximately 1–3 months later large numbers of hairs are shed as new hairs emerge. Anagen defluxion is a similar condition except that the large shed of hairs occurs shortly after (within days to a week) the event. Hairs from anagen defluxion often show a narrowing in the hair shaft or a sudden break. The sudden stressor causes a temporary cessation of hair growth manifested by a narrowing or weak spot in the growing hair.

ii. Treatment is not needed. The hair coat should regrow within 3–6 months.

iii. The five classifications are: immediate anagen release (anagen hairs prematurely enter telogen and hair loss starts in 3–5 weeks); delayed anagen release (hairs remain in anagen for longer than normal, and their release starts when hairs grow in 2–3 months); short anagen (idiopathic shortening of anagen results in increased shedding and decreased hair length); immediate telogen release (normal telogen is shortened and hair loss begins in days to weeks); and delayed telogen release (telogen is prolonged) (Headington, 1993; Scott *et al.*, 2001g).

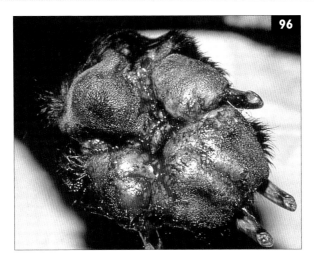

96 An adult (18-month-old) dog was presented for lameness and bleeding of the paws of 4 months' duration. The owner reported that the lesions developed slowly, and only recently did all four paws look similar to the one shown (96). The paws were painful, swollen, and exudative. The interdigital tissue was friable, and blood and pus exuded from the area when it was touched.

i. This is a case of pododermatitis. This is a clinical example of what type of pyoderma?

ii. What is the most common underlying cause of generalized pododermatitis in a dog of this age, and how is it treated? What is the most common cause of pododermatitis in dogs?

iii. What are sterile granuloma syndrome and nodular dermatofibrosis syndrome?

97 A cytological smear of ear exudate is made and cocci, rods, and peanut-shaped organisms are found. A culture and sensitivity of the exudate is requested.

i. What cocci are most commonly isolated from the ears of dogs?

ii.What rods are most commonly isolated from the ears of dogs with otitis?

iii.What is the most likely identity of the peanut-shaped organism?

96 i. Deep pyoderma. Blood, pus, and pain are the hallmarks of deep pyoderma. Patients are often febrile and have regional lymphadenopathy.

ii. Demodicosis. Because these patients are in much pain it can be difficult to do proper deep skin scrapings. Thus, *Demodex* mites can be missed in these patients. In other cases, mites can be hard to find due to chronic granulation tissue. If mites are suspected but not found, a skin biopsy should be done to eliminate demodicosis as a cause of deep pyoderma/pododermatitis.

The deep bacterial infection needs to be treated with an appropriate antibiotic; it cannot be stressed enough that treatment will require 4–12 weeks of oral antibiotics. Because therapy will be prolonged and expensive, a bacterial culture and sensitivity is recommended since often more than one pathogen is present. The dog needs to be treated for demodicosis. Amitraz therapy weekly is the initial treatment of choice. Whole body dips with concurrent foot soaks in amitraz are the author's first choice of treatment. It could be argued that ivermectin or milbemycin may be more appropriate in such cases because therapy could be started immediately and, as systemic agents, they may penetrate more readily into tissues. Often, the feet are the last region to clear of mites because of scar tissue, and the inability of amitraz to penetrate into tissues.

Unfortunately, many dogs with pododemodicosis cannot be cured. Dogs that fail amitraz therapy may respond to other therapies or may require maintenance miticidal therapy (e.g. amitraz) for life; treatment may vary from weekly to monthly depending upon the situation. In situations where chronic therapy is appropriate, the goal of therapy is to keep the patient lesion free even though the dog still shows positive skin scraping for mites. Dogs with generalized demodicosis should not be bred, as the tendency to develop this skin disease appears to be heritable.

iii. Sterile granuloma syndrome is an idiopathic disease that is common in many breeds, especially English bulldogs, great Dane dogs, boxers, and dachshunds. In this disorder, dogs develop nodular lesions particularly on their feet. The lesions are histologically pyogranulomatous but are negative for bacterial and fungal culture; hence the name. The pathogenesis is unknown. The disease is important to recognize because it can mimic bacterial pododermatitis, but it responds to glucocorticoid therapy. Nodular dermatofibrosis is primarily a disease of German shepherd dogs that presents clinically with nodular lesions on the feet and legs. The nodules are associated with renal cystadenomas or cystadenocarcinomas in both kidneys.

97 i. Gram-positive cocci, most likely to be *Staphylococcus intermedius* or *Streptococcus* spp.

ii. The most commonly isolated rods from the ear canal are *E. coli*, *Proteus*, *Klebsiella*, or *Pseudomonas* spp.

iii. Large peanut-shaped organisms are *Malassezia* spp.

98 A 9-month-old intact female Labrador retriever dog was referred for the complaint of persistent pruritus (98a, b). The owners practice flea control, and the other two dogs in the house are normal. The dog sleeps with the family's children, and none of them have skin lesions. The dog was treated for *Sarcoptes scabiei* mites with both lime sulfur (once weekly sponge-on dips for 6 weeks) and ivermectin (200 µg/kg PO every 2 weeks for 6 weeks). The pruritus

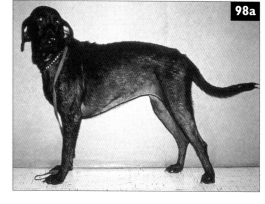

did not respond to a 4 week course of oral antibiotics (cephalexin) and ketoconazole at the appropriate dose and dosage for this patient. Skin scrapings, flea combings, and a dermatophyte culture were negative. The only other piece of historical information obtained was the owners reported the dog defecates 3–4 times a day, even though it is fed only once daily. The feces vary in consistency from firm to soft. Dermatological examination reveals hair lodged between the dog's teeth and gums, generalized thinning of the hair coat, and a mild oiliness to the coat.

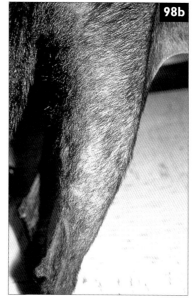

i. What differential diagnoses have been ruled out by the previous diagnostics?
ii. What are the most likely differential diagnoses at this time, and what diagnostic tests should be performed at this time?
iii. What is the relationship between intestinal parasitism and cutaneous pruritus?

99 What is piedra, what clinical signs does it cause, what other differential diagnoses must be considered, and what is the treatment of choice?

98, 99: Answers

98 i. The negative skin scrapings rule out demodicosis. The lime sulfur and ivermectin therapy rule out lice and *Sarcoptes* and *Cheyletiella* mites. In addition, these are highly contagious mites, and the other dogs in the house are normal, and the children have no symptoms. The negative fungal culture and 4 week treatment trial with antimicrobials rule out infections as a cause. The use of flea control makes a flea infestation or lice infestation unlikely, as well as FAD. Also, the distribution of clinical signs is inconsistent with classical FAD.

ii. The most likely differential diagnoses are food allergy and/or atopy. The frequent bowel movements could be related to the skin disease, since some dogs with food allergies have concurrent colitis. Owners may report that the dog strains and/or defecates several times a day. This dog could also have intestinal parasites and be suffering from a poorly understood disease called intestinal parasite hypersensitivity. Finally, this dog is an intact female, and another poorly understood disease called hormonal hypersensitivity could be the cause of the pruritus. A direct fecal smear and a fecal flotation should be done to rule out intestinal parasites. If necessary, the dog should be treated with an appropriate anthelmintic. If this dog has intestinal parasite hypersensitivity, the pruritus will resolve with treatment. Surgical neutering should be discussed with the owners, not only because estrus cycles are a possible (but rare) cause of pruritus, but also for the obvious health benefits for the dog. In addition, the most obvious dermatological test to pursue is a restricted food trial for up to 12 weeks. The food trial should be delayed until after the dog has recovered from surgery. Although most commercial or home cooked diets are formulated to be complete and balanced, they may not contain enough calories and protein for a patient recovering from surgery. If the food trial is negative, or if there is only a partial response, the dog should be evaluated for atopy. This dog was diagnosed with a food allergy to beef and remained symptom free as long as she was fed a beef- and beef by-product-free dog food.

iii. The intestinal mucosa is a protective barrier that does not permit antigens to cross into the body. It has been proposed that one of the mechanisms by which dogs become sensitized to various food antigens is via a damaged mucosal barrier. Intestinal parasites (round worms, hookworms, and tape worms) damage the mucosal barrier and allow antigens into the submucosa, leading to sensitization. In addition, viral diseases of the gut are believed to play a similar role in predisposing animals to food allergies.

99 Piedra is an uncommon fungal infection of the hair shaft. It is caused by one of two organisms, *Piedraia hortae* or *Trichosporon biegelii*. These infections are usually asymptomatic and present as nodular lesions on the hair shaft. Differential diagnoses include trihorrhexis nodosa, trihomycosis axillaries, hair casts, and abnormal hair shaft development. These infections are usually self-limiting and shaving of the hair coat and topical antimycotic shampoo therapy is usually curative.

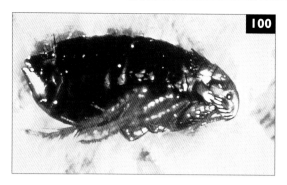

100 What is this parasite (100)?

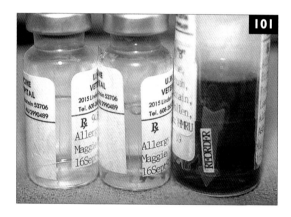

101 The illustration shows three vials of a new immunotherapy prescription for a patient (101).

i. Two of the vials are dilutions of the concentrated or maintenance vial (Vial 3). Why are dilutions made and administered to patients?

ii. What is the 'correct' injection schedule for administration of the allergen, and how should the allergen be stored?

iii. How long will it take before the patient shows maximal benefit from allergen immunotherapy? Assuming the patient shows benefit from the therapy, how long will the patient need to receive the immunotherapy?

100 *Ctenocephalides felis*, adult cat flea.

101 i. The individual stock allergens purchased from an allergy company range in concentration from 20,000–40,00 PNU/ml. The maintenance vial consists of an individualized mixture of allergens for each patient and is made from the commercial stock solutions and varies in concentration from 20,000–40,000 PNU/ml. It is too concentrated and patients are at risk of localized or generalized anaphylaxis if it is administered without an induction period. Two 1:10 serial dilutions are made from the patient's maintenance vial (Vial 2, 2000–4000 PNU/ml; and Vial 1, 200–400 PNU/ml). Immunotherapy injections are administered subcutaneously. Patients receive increasing volumes of Vial 1 every 2–3 days until a total volume of 1 ml is administered. At that time, Vial 1 is discarded and small increasing volumes of Vial 2 are administered until the patient has received a total of 1 ml. This process is repeated until the patient is receiving 1 ml of Vial 3.
ii. There is no one correct injection schedule. All schedules are tailored to the patient's response to therapy. The initial phase of therapy takes about 30 days to complete. After this, the patient receives a maintenance injection at regular intervals; the time interval between injections is tailored to the patient and may vary from 7–10 days to every 21 days. The optimum interval between injections is determined by recording the severity of pruritus between injections. For example, if a patient is receiving a maintenance injection every 10 days but becomes pruritic after day 8, the appropriate interval between injections is about 8 days. The target volume of 1 ml is also not absolute. Patients that develop pruritus shortly after the administration of 1 ml of allergen, may not be able to tolerate this much allergen. In these cases, a decrease in the volume (e.g. 0.75 ml instead of 1 ml) may be beneficial. On occasion, Vial 3 is too concentrated and a patient's maintenance vial is Vial 2 (2000–4000 PNU/ml).
Allergens should be refrigerated to prevent premature degradation of allergen proteins and to prevent bacterial contamination. The allergen liquid is a clear amber color. Cloudy vials or vials with flocculent material indicate bacterial contamination. The most common cause of bacterial contamination is a client that reuses needles and/or does not refrigerate the allergen.
iii. Immunotherapy is beneficial in the treatment of atopy in both dogs and cats in approximately 70% of cases. In general, patients can start to show signs of benefit anywhere between 3 and 12 months of therapy. Immunotherapy is generally considered to be life-long therapy. Therefore, it is important to select patients carefully for this type of therapy. Seasonally atopic patients are usually managed medically. As a rule of thumb, the best candidates for immunotherapy are patients with severe seasonal allergies, year round allergies, patients that do not respond to medical therapy, or patients with concurrent medical conditions that preclude the use of glucocorticoids (e.g. diabetes mellitus).

102 One of five cats in a multi-cat household is presented as an emergency. One week prior to presentation the owner found a small amount of blood on the cat's face. Today the cat is febrile (40°C [105°F]), depressed, has hair loss, and an open wound on the side of its face (102).

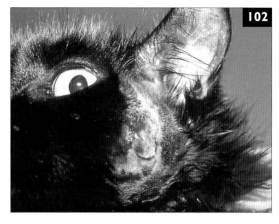

i. What is the most likely diagnosis, how should it be confirmed, and how should it be treated?

ii. Three weeks later the owner presents the same cat for examination. The owner reports that the cat's skin lesion showed only a partial response to treatment. What diseases should be considered at this time?

iii. What is CSD?

103 A 12-year-old cat is presented for the sudden development of greasy seborrhea (103). The cat is nonpruritic, there are no other inflammatory skin lesions found on physical examination, and the cat has no previous history of skin disease. The owner reports the cat has stopped grooming itself and has lost weight. Oily seborrhea is uncommon in cats, especially in older cats. What non-dermatological diseases should be investigated for in this cat?

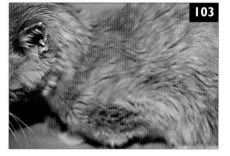

102 i. Cat bite abscess. The blood was the result of a bite or claw wound from a housemate. Cat bite abscesses are common in cats that go outdoors and/or that live in multi-cat households. Lesions are found on the face, shoulders, tail base, paws, and inguinal areas. This is usually a clinical diagnosis. The most commonly isolated pathogen is *Pasteurella multocida*. Other organisms commonly found in the oral cavity may be cultured. Although more difficult to culture, anaerobes are more commonly isolated than aerobic bacteria. Cytological findings would compatible with septic inflammation: inter- and intracellular bacteria would most likely be found.

The cat should be sedated, the hair coat from the wound should be clipped, the wound surgically drained, explored for a possible foreign body, and the wound flushed with saline or chlorhexidine solution. Antibiotic therapy alone is likely to fail in cases where the lesion is not drained. Systemic antibiotic therapy for 1–2 weeks is most commonly prescribed, especially in cats that are depressed and febrile. *Pasteurella multocida* is susceptible to penicillin antibiotics.

ii. The medical problem at this point is a non-healing wound. It is still possible that this is due to the original cat bite abscess; there could be a walled-off area of sequestered infection. Differential diagnoses include: sporotrichosis, foreign body, *Cuterebra* larva, and *Nocardia* or mycobacterial infection. *Gloves should always be worn and lesions should be considered of zoonotic/infectious origin until proven otherwise.*

iii. CSD is a zoonotic bacterial infection caused by *Bartonella henselae* (Breitschwerdt and Greene, 1998). These bacteria are fastidious, arthropod-transmitted organisms and cats appear to be the reservoir of infection. The disease can be transmitted to people via cat bites, cat saliva, or bites from fleas or ticks feeding on infected cats. In cats, this disease is considered to be a self-limiting febrile illness of 48–72 hours. Some animals will develop neurological symptoms, anorexia, and peripheral lymph-adenopathy. Most infections in cats, however, are subclinical. The disease in people is associated with a variety of syndromes but is highly dependent upon the immune status of the individual. This is one of the reasons why routine and consistent flea and tick control are recommended for cats.

103 Greasy seborrhea is very rare in the cat, and when it happens it should be considered a dermatological sign of a systemic disease: liver, pancreatic, or intestinal disease, drug eruptions, systemic lupus erythematosus, hyperthyroidism, diabetes mellitus, FeLV or FIV, and neoplasia. This was a case of greasy seborrhea secondary to feline hyperthyroidism. The greasy seborrhea seen in feline patients with these diseases is most likely due to poor grooming on the part of the cat and not a direct relationship between the disease and the skin.

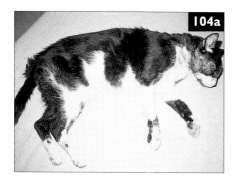
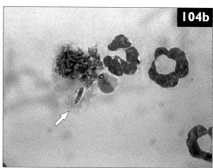

104 A second opinion is requested on a cat with nonhealing wounds on the face and limbs for 6 weeks. Another veterinarian diagnosed cat bite abscess and prescribed 21 days of oral antibiotics at the correct dose and dosage. The cat did not respond, and the owner reports the infection seems to be spreading. On physical examination, a severe ulcerative lesion on the face is noted and numerous smaller lesions on the inner forelegs (104a). Exudate for bacterial and fungal culture is collected and an impression smear of the exudate performed. The impression smear shows severe neutrophilic inflammation and numerous intracytoplasmic organisms (104b, arrow).
i. What is the diagnosis, and what is the treatment of choice?
ii. Where can dogs and cats acquire this disease?
iii. What are the public health considerations?

105 This dog was presented for pruritus (105). Note the hair loss over the dorsum and along the caudal thighs. Skin scrapings and a fungal culture were negative. Flea combings were negative for fleas, flea excreta, lice, or *Cheyletiella* mites. The dog's pruritus had not responded to antimicrobial therapy.
i. What is the most likely diagnosis given the information provided?
ii. What is the treatment for this condition?
iii. How does the condition develop and what immunological reactions are involved?

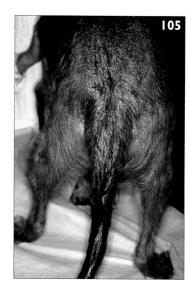

104 i. *Sporothrix schenckii.* Note the cigar-shaped organism surrounded by a clear space. In cats, nonhealing wounds are a common clinical presentation of this intermediate fungal disease. Organisms are plentiful on cytological preparations in cats, but not in dogs. Itraconazole (5–10 mg/kg PO q24h) is the treatment of choice, and treatment should be continued for at least 30 days past clinical cure. Cats often require 4–8 weeks of treatment.

ii. Sporotrichosis is a subcutaneous fungal disease caused by a dimorphic fungus, *Sporothrix schenckii.* The organism is found worldwide and grows as a saprophyte in the soil and in dead organic debris. It is also found in barberry and rose bush thorns, sphagnum moss, tree bark, and timber. Outbreaks of the disease have been associated with sphagnum moss used in horticulture to pack seedlings, young trees, and hanging decorative flower baskets. The organism does not grow on living moss but rather on dead decaying moss (Zhang and Andrews, 1993). The handling of stored bales of hay has also been associated with disease (Rosser and Dunstan, 1998).

iii. This is a zoonotic disease; however, people can and often do contract it spontaneously from the environment. Cases of cat-to-people transmission have been primarily limited to veterinary health care workers coming into contact with infected exudate. In some instances, infection has occurred after nontraumatic exposure, suggesting that the cat form is particularly virulent and can gain entry into the skin through microscopic breaks. People handling cats with abscesses should wear disposable gloves and thoroughly wash their hand and arms with chlorhexidine or povidone-iodine scrubs.

105 i. Fleas and/or FAD. This is a classic distribution for flea infestations or flea allergy in dogs. FAD is a hypersensitivity to the bite of the flea, and it is common to find a low number of fleas in these animals.

ii. The management of FAD in dogs requires the identification and treatment of secondary bacterial and/or yeast infections, consistent and thorough flea control on the pet and in the home, and the alleviation of pruritus. The latter may be complicated by the presence of secondary infections. Glucocorticoids are contraindicated if secondary infections are present.

iii. FAD can be experimentally induced in dogs by intermittent flea exposure. In one study, dogs were exposed once weekly for 15 minutes to fleas and within 40 weeks developed clinical signs of FAD when challenged with flea infestations (Halliwell, 1990). Dogs that were continuously exposed to fleas developed tolerance to fleas and a delayed onset of hypersensitivity. This work suggests that intermittent exposure to fleas is an important trigger in the development of FAD. The immune reactions to fleas are complex. Intradermal skin testing with flea antigen demonstrated that there is an immediate, late phase (basophil influx), and delayed or cell-mediated response to this arthropod.

106 A raised solitary lesion is shown on the lower eyelid of a 3-year-old cat (106). The owner reported that the lesion had been present for several months. Previously, another veterinarian told her that it was an 'eyelid cyst'. Except for this lesion, the cat is otherwise healthy. Cats do not often develop infections of the sebaceous glands of the eyelids (meibomian styes or hordeolums), and the lesion is suspicious and

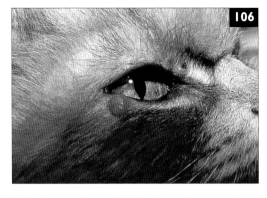

may be a mast cell tumor. A FNA of the lesion confirms this. The lesion is excised, and the diagnosis is confirmed. A buffy coat smear is negative for mast cells.

i. What is the prognosis for this cat?
ii. What is the behavior of ocular or eyelid melanomas in the cat?
iii. What is DNA ploidy?

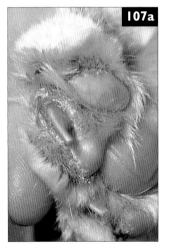
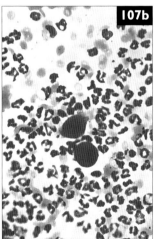

107 A cat was presented for lameness. Note the swollen skin around the base of the nails (107a).

i. What is this condition called, and what are the most common causes of this condition in the cat?
ii. What diagnostic tests are indicated?
iii. A smear of the exudate from the nail bed is shown (107b). How could these findings be described, and what is the most likely diagnosis?

106 i. The prognosis for a cat with a solitary lesion is good. In cats, the vast majority of cutaneous MCT are benign. The cat should be monitored for recurrence and/or development of new lesions. Most feline MCT occur on the head and neck, and even with a histologically incomplete excision most do not recur. Multiple tumors with a generalized distribution over the body are more likely to be associated with malignant biological behavior (i.e. spread to other sites and/or organs) than solitary tumors. Cutaneous MCT can also represent metastatic lesions from visceral forms of the disease, which carry a worse prognosis.

ii. Most melanomas in the cat involve the eye or the eyelid. Unlike the situation in the dog, histological assessment of malignancy does not predict the clinical behavior. Ocular melanomas are behaviorally more malignant than oral melanomas, and dermal melanomas are most likely to have a benign course in the cat.

iii. DNA ploidy refers to the cellular DNA content, where diploid means normal DNA content, and aneuploid means abnormal (either increased or decreased) DNA content. It is measured by flow cytometry, which is a rapid and precise measurement of DNA ploidy and the distribution of the cell cycle phases (G_0, G_1, G_2, and M) of a tissue sample. This is a very important tool because it can rapidly measure hundreds of thousands of cells, help to determine prognosis, and clarify the distinction between high- and low-risk tumors. In the case of melanomas, DNA ploidy was found to be no more predictive than simple light microscopy and is not considered cost effective (Bolon *et al.*, 1990).

107 i. Paronychia. The most common causes of paronychia in the cat are trauma, dermatophytosis, *Malassezia* dermatitis, demodicosis, *Notoedres* mites, and PF.

ii. A Wood's lamp examination is optional, but a dermatophyte culture should be prepared. Exudate from the nail base should be collected, smeared on a glass microscope slide, heat fixed, and stained. *Malassezia* dermatitis is an under-recognized skin disease in cats, and the most common presentation is an accumulation of black debris under the nail. Bacterial culture and sensitivity should also be done, along with a skin scraping using mineral oil to look for mites. A skin biopsy may be needed for a definitive diagnosis.

iii. There is neutrophilic inflammatory exudate with large basophilic epithelial cells. These cells are compatible with what would be described as 'acantholytic cells' (**107b**). These are epidermal cells from the stratum spinosum that have been shed into the pustular exudate. These cells are often seen in patients with PF and in patients with severe deep pyoderma. In PF, the cells are usually very numerous and often present in rafts of 6–8 cells. In patients with deep pyoderma, the number of cells adhered together are fewer, often just two or three. This was a case of paronychia due to a *Microsporum canis* infection.

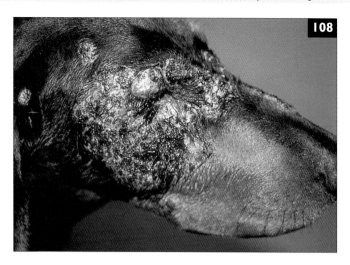

108 A 3-year-old male doberman pinscher dog was presented for examination because the lesions depicted did not respond to oral antibiotics (cephalexin 30 mg/kg PO q12h for 21 days); the owner self-medicated the dog. Upon further questioning, the owner stated that the lesion started out as a small raised nodule and, over the course of 5–6 weeks, developed into a severely proliferative and exudative lesion (108). The dog was mildly febrile, had weight loss, and bilateral corneal ulcerations. Impression smears of the exudates were consistent with septic inflammation. Anaerobic and aerobic bacterial cultures and fungal culture were performed.
i. What other diagnostic test is indicated?
ii. What differential diagnoses should the pathologist be told are being considered?
iii. Cats rarely develop this type of lesion. However, something similar has been described in longhaired cats. Elaborate.

109 What are the treatment options for canine hyperadrenocorticism?

108 i. Skin biopsy. Numerous skin biopsy specimens should be taken from various sites on the lesion. It is important NOT to scrub or wipe the target sample sites prior to the biopsy. In some sites, a skin biopsy punch instrument would be suitable. However, if the tissue is very thickened, a deep wedge biopsy using a scalpel blade is recommended.
ii. The pathologist should be provided with a complete history. It is important to include information about previous diagnostic tests (lack of response to antibiotic therapy, negative bacterial and fungal cultures) because this will help the pathologist decide which, if any, special stains may be needed. The considered differential diagnoses in this case include neoplasia, deep fungal infections, dermatophyte kerion reaction, mycetoma, and phaeohyphomycosis. All of these differentials can look similar and are differentiated based upon histological examination of tissues.
A kerion reaction is an exudative inflammatory reaction to dermatophytes. It is most commonly seen with *Microsporum gypseum* or *Trichophyton mentagrophytes*. A mycetoma is a subcutaneous skin infection in which tissue grains are present. These 'grains' are believed to be composed of the infectious agent and/or antigen–antibody response. Mycetomas are caused by fungi (eumycotic mycetomas) or bacteria such as *Actinomyces* or *Nocardia*. Phaeohyphomycosis is another subcutaneous fungal infection caused by pigmented or dematiaceous fungi. It differs from a mycetoma in that tissue grains are not present. This dog had a diffuse fungal kerion reaction due to *T. mentagrophytes*. The bacterial culture was negative, and the initial fungal culture was also negative. After receiving the biopsy report and noting the presence of dermatophytes and a kerion reaction, a fungal culture from the peripheral region of the lesion was obtained, and *T. mentagrophytes* was isolated. This dog lived on a small farm, and the owner had several hobby cattle and horses. Thus, the source of exposure was presumed to be the large animals. The patient responded to 5 weeks of oral griseofulvin therapy.
iii. The acute onset and rapid spread of the lesion in this dog, along with the history suggests that this may be kerion reaction to a dermatophyte. In cats, kerion reactions are uncommon. Granulomatous dermatitis has been described in longhaired cats. Affected cats developed subcutaneous nodules, and in one case, disseminated disease from *M. canis*. This has been called *M. canis* pseudomycetoma or more appropriately, fungal granuloma. Other names have included mycetoma or Majocchi's granuloma. These lesions occur on cats with generalized dermatophytosis, and in one case, the strain of *M. canis* isolated from the skin was different than the one isolated from the tumor. Treatment is difficult and surgical excision and long-term itraconazole have been effective.

109 Adrenalectomy is the treatment of choice for adrenal tumors. Pituitary-dependent adrenal hyperplasia is most commonly treated with mitotane. Alternative therapies include ketoconazole, selegiline, and trilostane.

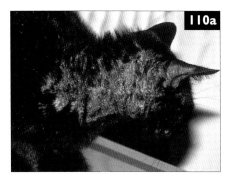
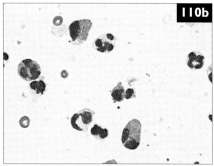

110 A cat was presented for 'bumpy skin' and pruritus of the head and neck (110a). Physical examination was normal except for the skin. Diffuse, small papular-crusted eruptions were present, primarily on the neck. The cat was an indoor-outdoor cat, and the owners did not practice flea control. Skin scrapings were negative. Flea combings of the trunk were negative for fleas and flea feces; however, fleas were noted on the cat's face. Impression smears of the skin were consistent with eosiniophilic inflammation (110b).
i. What is the clinical term for this cat's 'bumpy skin'? What differential diagnoses should be considered?
ii. What is the initial treatment plan?
iii. The owner is a concerned the cat may have hypereosinophilic syndrome. What are the clinical signs of this disease?

111 A 6-month old Siamese cat with multiple cutaneous nodules on its head, face, and ears is presented for examination (111). Skin biopsy findings reveal a histiocytic MCT.
i. What is the cat's prognosis?
ii. What are the three major clinical presentations of MCT in cats?
iii. What are the two histological subtypes of cutaneous MCT in cats?

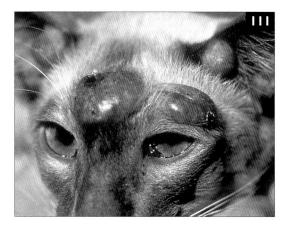

110 i. Miliary dermatitis. This is one of many eosinophilic reaction patterns in cats, but note this is not a diagnosis but rather a clinical sign. These lesions are often found more easily upon palpation of the skin rather than on visual examination. This reaction pattern is most commonly seen in parasitic infestations, bacterial and fungal infections, food allergy, atopy, and FAD. In this case, the most likely cause is flea infestation/FAD.
ii. Initial treatment should be directed at treating the cat for FAD. Flea control for this cat and all other animals in the household should be prescribed. The monthly spot-on flea control products would be ideal for this indoor-outdoor cat. A subcutaneous injection of methlyprednisone (20 mg/cat) could be administered to alleviate the pruritus and resolve the skin lesions. Treatment may need to be repeated. It is important to follow-up on this patient to determine if flea control alone eventually controls the symptoms. If not, then food allergy and/or atopy should be investigated.
iii. Hypereosinophilic syndrome is a rare disease characterized by idiopathic eosinophilia that infiltrates various tissues. Although a macular–papular eruption on the skin can occur, it is rare. The most common clinical signs are diarrhea, weight loss, vomiting, and anorexia. Thickened bowel loops, lymphadenopathy, hepatomegaly, and splenomegaly are also common.

111 i. The prognosis is good. These tumors in young Siamese cats (<4 years of age) usually undergo spontaneous remission. These lesions also can be seen in non-Siamese kittens and will also resolve spontaneously. Adult cats of other breeds with widespread lesions should be evaluated carefully as these cats tend to have visceral involvement.
ii. The three forms of clinical presentation are cutaneous, lymphoreticular or visceral, and gastrointestinal. The visceral form involves a combination of the liver, spleen and/or abdominal lymph nodes. The cutaneous form is limited to the skin. The gastrointestinal form is usually a primary tumor and is the third most common intestinal tumor in cats after lymphoma and adenocarcinoma (Thamm and Vail, 2001). These tumors usually arise from the small intestine. Eosinophilia may be present. Clinical signs of lymphoreticular and gastrointestinal MCTs are indistinguishable: vomiting, diarrhea, depression, weight loss, and anorexia.
iii. The two histological subtypes of feline mast cells are the histiocytic and mast cell type. The histiocytic type occurs in young cats (<4 years of age) and is most common in Siamese cats. It frequently presents as subcutaneous nodules. Histologically, the mast cells are poorly granulated and lymphoid aggregates are common. Many of these tumors will spontaneously regress. The 'mast cell form' of cutaneous MCT tends to occur in mixed breed shorthaired cats. Lesions tend to be solitary and are discrete, nodular, papular, or plaque-like lesions in the dermis or subcutaneous tissue. It can also present as 'miliary dermatitis'.

112 An intensely pruritic dog was presented for examination. The dog's pruritus developed acutely approximately 3 weeks ago. The dog had no history of skin disease prior to this episode. The dog was normal on physical examination except for being intensely pruritic and having 'scaly' elbows (112a). The organism shown was found on a skin scraping from the elbow of the patient (112b).

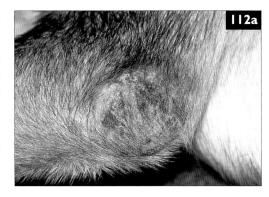

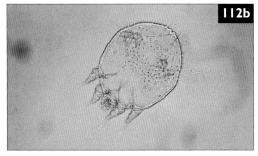

i. What is the organism?

ii. What clinical signs are associated with this parasite infestation?

iii. What new diagnostic test is available, and what are the limitations of the test?

113 A neutered female cat was presented for the problem of 'tail fungus'. The cat's dorsal tail region was mildly pruritic, waxy, and matted (113). The cat was otherwise normal. When the owner was asked why she thought the cat had a fungal infection, she said the area 'glowed' when examined with a Wood's lamp.

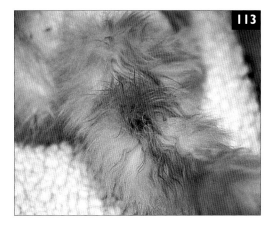

i. This is a very common skin disorder found on the tail of cats. What is it, and how is it treated?

ii. Why did the area glow when exposed to a Wood's lamp?

iii. What husbandry practices contribute to this problem?

112, 113: Answers

112 i. *Sarcoptes scabiei* mite.

ii. This is a highly contagious mite that causes intense pruritus. The history of an acute onset of intense pruritus is common. The mites burrow in thinly haired areas, and intense ventral pruritus may be the first clinical sign noted. In many cases, there is a history of exposure to affected dogs or high-risk exposure situations (e.g. stray dogs, boarding kennel, visit to a grooming facility, visit to a park). In many patients, lesions may be absent but thinly haired areas, the ventrum, elbows, and ear margins, are often good sites to find mites. Both deep and superficial skin scrapings should be done to increase the chances of finding the mites.

iii. Recently, an *in vitro* serum antibody test was marketed in Sweden for the diagnosis of this parasite. The test is reported to have a sensitivity of 83% and a specificity of 92% (Curtis, 2001).

113 i. Dorsal tail seborrhea or hyperplasia. The common lay term for this condition is 'stud tail'. This is a disorder of keratinization caused by excessive oil and sebum production. The dorsal surface of the tail of cats contains large numbers of sebaceous glands, and in some cats they become overactive and exudate accumulates on the dorsal surface. This condition can occur in both female and male cats, regardless of whether or not they have been neutered. Castration will not resolve the problem.

Impression smears of the oily material should be obtained to look for secondary yeast or bacterial skin infections, especially if the cat is pruritic. Secondary *Malassezia* infections are common. If secondary infections are found, they should be treated for 21–30 days with appropriate antimicrobial drugs (e.g. cephalexin or itraconazole). Topical, daily washings with an antifungal shampoo (ketoconazole, miconazole) is another treatment option for yeast infections. The treatment of choice for the waxy debris is frequent bathing of the tail area with a cleansing shampoo (e.g. a flea shampoo) or a mild antiseborrheic shampoo. Treatment is usually life-long unless the cat resumes normal grooming.

ii. The fluorescence is caused by the accumulation of sebum (skin oils) on the skin and hair. Sebum commonly glows when exposed to an ultraviolet light or Wood's lamp (e.g. chin and tail areas). The color of the fluorescence varies and is a known cause of false positive Wood's lamp examinations. True fluorescence is apple green in color. Diagnosis should be limited to the hairs since sebum on the skin surface will glow, giving a false positive.

iii. Tail gland hyperplasia and excessive oily seborrhea are more common in cats that are confined to small spaces and/or facilities with multiple cats. Cats confined to small spaces and/or stressed by overcrowding may not groom properly. In addition, this condition may develop in cats that are unable to groom properly, including obese, elderly, arthritic, and/or injured cats.

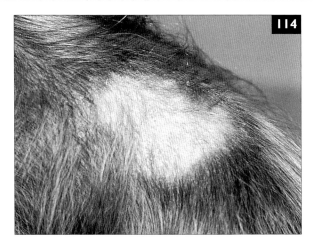

114 In January, a 1-year-old dog is presented for treatment of 'ringworm'. The owner reports the dog has developed a 'ringworm' lesion on its dorsal back. There are two other dogs in the house along with three indoor cats, and none of these animals show signs of skin disease. The dog in question sleeps with the owner and she doesn't have skin lesions. Dermatological examination reveals a focal area of noninflammatory hair loss (114) in the right lateral lumbosacral area. A Wood's lamp examination is negative. The medical record indicates the dog received a subcutaneous injection of glucocorticoids 3.5 months ago at the end of September for seasonal atopy. The location of the injection was recorded as 'subcutaneous over on the dorsum'. The dog is frequently groomed, and the owner has a penchant for having ribbons braided into the dog's hair coat.

i. What are the most common differential diagnoses for acquired noninflammatory focal alopecia, and what diagnostic tests should be performed?

ii. The skin biopsy findings revealed a focal area of thinning of the dermis and epidermis and atrophy of the hair follicles. What is the most likely diagnosis, and what management recommendations should be made?

iii. List the major etiologies that cause focal damage to hair follicles and give at least one disease example in each category.

115 A dog with severe *Pseudomonas* otitis media is to be treated with ticarcillin (Timentin®) otitic solution, compounded from the injectable formulation. 20 ml of a 20 mg/ml concentration is required. Timentin® is supplied in a 3.1 g vial. The package says to reconstitute the drug by adding 13 ml of sterile water to yield a concentration of 200 mg/ml. How should this prescription be compounded?

114 i. Differential diagnoses include alopecia areata, traction alopecia, post-rabies vaccination alopecia, and post-glucocorticoid injection site alopecia. The anti-inflammatory effects of glucocorticoids could be masking the inflammation usually associated with an infectious disease such as pyoderma, demodicosis, or dermato-phytosis, and these should be included in the differential diagnoses. Traction alopecia is a clinical syndrome seen in small breed dogs that have ribbons, barrettes, or bows tied too tightly into their hair coat. The tension on the hair follicles results in damage to the vasculature and permanent loss of hair follicles. Subcutaneous rabies vaccina-tions can cause vasculitis and a focal area of alopecia at the site of injection. Topical and subcutaneous glucocorticoids are also associated with focal areas of alopecia. The most useful diagnostic tests include skin scrapings, impression smears, dermatophyte cultures, and a skin biopsy. These tests were normal or negative.
ii. The skin biopsy findings were interpreted as compatible with an endocrine alopecia. This was a case of post-steroid injection alopecia. The dog's hair regrew over the next 6 months, and the lesion recurred in the fall when the dog again received a gluco-corticoid injection. Post-injection hair loss is a possible side-effect of repositol glucocorticoids, and owners should be warned that hair loss could occur at the site.
iii. Follicular infections (bacteria, yeast, and dermatophytes), follicular parasites (demodicosis), nutritional diseases (zinc deficiency), neoplasia (epitheliotrophic lymphoma), immune-mediated diseases (pemphigus, sebaceous adenitis, alopcecia areata), and trauma (burns, vascular damage, i.e. traction alopecia, dermatomyositis) (Paterson, 2002).

115 Reconstituting the drug by adding 13 ml of sterile water yields a concentration of 200 mg/ml (3.1 g ÷ [13 ml water + 2.5 ml powder volume]).

First, calculate the number of mg of Timentin® needed in 20 ml:
   20 mg/ml × 20 ml = 400 mg

Next, calculate how many ml of Timentin® 200 mg/ml is needed to get that amount:
   400 mg ÷ 200 mg/ml = 2 ml of Timentin® 200 mg/ml

Then, calculate the quantity of NaCl 0.9% to add to obtain a 20 ml solution of Timentin® 20 mg/ml:
   20 ml – 2 ml = 18 ml of NaCl 0.9%

Note: This solution is commonly used by the author for the treatment of resistant *Pseudomonas* strains. The remaining stock solution (200 mg/ml) can be frozen in aliquots of 2 ml for future use.

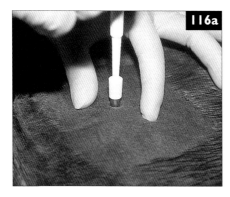

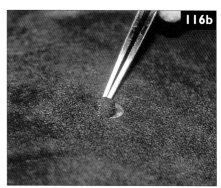

116 Skin biopsies are very important diagnostic tests in veterinary dermatology. The illustrations show key steps in the collection of samples where sample handling can cause distortion and artifacts.
i. How can creating artifacts be avoided when selecting and preparing a site for sampling?
ii. How can creating artifacts be avoided when using a skin biopsy punch (116a)?
iii. How can creating artifacts be avoided when handling the specimen collected with a skin biopsy punch (116b, c)?

117 A 5-year-old female poodle dog was presented for the complaint of anal licking and scooting. The owner reported that the problem started about 4 weeks ago after they returned from their winter vacation to Florida. Physical examination revealed salivary staining of the skin around the anus and a mildly erythematous perineal area. Rectal examination revealed mildly filled anal sacs that were difficult to express; the secretion was thick and tan in color.
i. What are the differential diagnoses?
ii. What is the immediate diagnostic and/or treatment plan?

116, 117: Answers

116 i. The most common causes of artifacts during sample site selection and preparation are damage of surface or target lesions with electric clipper blades, surgical preparation of the site, and inadvertent intradermal injection of lidocaine. The hair coat should be clipped very carefully or with scissors to prevent damage of the site. The biopsy site SHOULD NOT be scrubbed or wiped prior to collection of the specimens. Finally, care needs to be taken to ensure that lidocaine is administered subcutaneously and not intradermally.

ii. The skin biopsy punch should be placed directly over the lesion. The skin on either side of the sample should be tensed to prevent shearing of the sample (**116a**). Once the punch has been placed, it should be pressed onto the skin gently but firmly, and rotated in one direction to prevent shearing and artifacts, until the sample is 'free'. Except where the skin is very thin, the biopsy specimen will be free from surrounding attachments when the skin biopsy reaches the hub of the punch.

iii. It is very important not to crush the sample when freeing it from the skin. In order to prevent this artifact, small forceps should be used to grasp gently the subcutaneous stack of the specimen and gently lift it up (**116b**). In many cases, this alone will free the specimen from the body. If not, a scalpel blade should be used to cut the subcutaneous tissue and free the specimen from the skin (**116c**).

117 i. Impacted anal sacs with or without secondary infection or pruritus ani resulting in secondary anal sac disease. Anal sac problems are more common in smaller breed dogs, especially obese dogs. Licking and scooting are suggestive of anal sac impactions or anal pruritus. It is possible that the dog became infested with fleas and subsequently tapeworms, as a result of the trip to Florida. Tapeworm segments can sometimes be found in anal sac expressions, fecal examinations, and/or on rectal examination. Many dogs with allergic skin disease (atopy, food allergy, contact allergy), vulvar fold dermatitis, vaginitis, tail fold dermatitis and prostate disease will develop pruritus ani. The resulting inflammation of the anal area causes the anal sac ducts to become narrowed leading to anal sac impactions, and possibly infection.

ii. Manual expression of the anal sacs is recommended. The secretion should be examined cytologically for evidence of infection and infectious agents (bacteria, and/or *Malassezia*). If there is evidence of infection, the anal sacs should be filled with an antimicrobial solution that contains a glucocorticoid. This should be repeated every 5–7 days. Alternatively, systemic antimicrobials (author's preference) can be administered for 14–21 days. A topical glucocorticoid can still be instilled into the sacs or the owner can apply a topical steroid to the perineal area. In this case, flea control should be discussed with the owners and prophylactic deworming for tapeworms should be considered. Surgical removal of the anal sacs will not resolve the anal pruritus if there is an underlying pruritic cause.

118 A 10-year-old DSH tabby cat is presented for the complaint of a 'bump' on the nose (**118a**). The owner reports that the lesion began as a scab, and it has been gradually enlarging. The cat also has had a chronic nasal discharge of several months duration. The cat is an indoor-outdoor and lives in the southwestern region of the USA. There is a mild purulent nasal discharge, and the nose is distorted. The 'bump' is rather firm on pal- pation. The cat is otherwise healthy on examination.

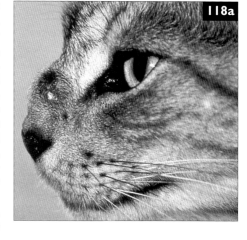

i. Given the history and clinical signs, what is the most probable cause of the lesion and nasal discharge?

ii. What diagnostics are indicated to confirm the diagnosis?

iii. What drugs have been used successfully to treat this disease in cats, how can therapy be monitored, and can the owner be given a prognosis?

119 A 3-year-old dog is shown (**119**).

i. This is a classic presentation of what allergic skin disease?

ii. How is this disease treated?

iii. What immunological mechanisms are believe to be involved in the development of this disease?

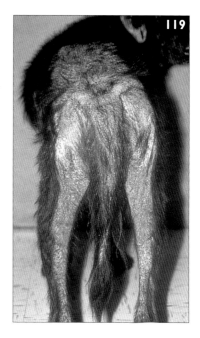

118 i. Feline cryptococcosis. This is a deep fungal disease caused by *Crypto-coccus neoformans*, a ubiquitous yeast-like fungus commonly associated with pigeon feces. This organism has a worldwide distribution and is the most common deep mycosis of cats. Upper respiratory signs, especially chronic nasal discharge and masses over the bridge of the nose are the most common clinical signs, but skin lesions are present in about 50% of cases. Cats

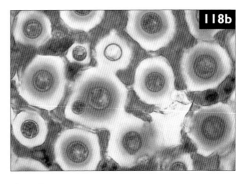

can also develop central nervous system and ocular signs.

ii. Definitive diagnosis can be made by finding the organism on cytological examination of nasal swabs, nasal flushes, and/or impression smears of exudates. The organism can also be found on biopsy; however, in this case, skin biopsy did not reveal the organism, and a nasal flush was needed to isolate the organism. The latex agglutination test can give false negative results in cats with only skin lesions. The organism (**118b**) is a round to elliptical 2–20 μm yeast-like organism, and has a mucinous capsule that produces a 'halo' around the organism.

iii. In some cases surgical debulking may be helpful when masses are large and/or are obstructing nasal passages. Cats have been successfully treated with amphotericin B, ketoconazole, itraconazole, and fluconazole; however, amphotericin B and keto-conazole are not well tolerated by cats. Itraconazole treatment is long (>8.5 months), the dose is high (20 mg/kg PO daily), and long-term therapy is associated with hepatotoxicity. Fluconazole is similar to itraconazole, and it is widely distributed and penetrates the blood–brain barrier.

Serial serum titers can be used to monitor response to therapy. Progressive decreases in serum antigen titers of at least 10-fold over 2 months suggest a favorable prognosis.

119 i. This is a classic case of FAD.

ii. FAD is treated with flea control. This patient has clinical signs of a secondary bacterial pyoderma (note the erythema on the hind legs). The dog should be treated with an appropriate course of antimicrobial therapy for a minimum of 4 weeks. Glucocorticoids should not be used in this patient to alleviate the pruritus until the microbial infections resolve, and the owner has initiated flea control. Immunotherapy for flea bite hypersensitivity has not been successful.

iii. The pruritus of FAD is believed to be caused by a combination of type 1, type 4, late phase reactions, and basophil hypersensitivity reactions.

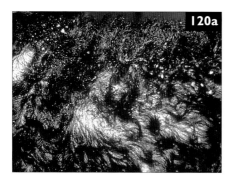

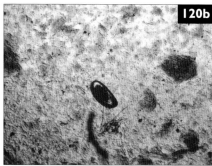

120 A 9-year-old black poodle dog with primary idiopathic seborrhea is presented for a second opinion (120a). The owner reports that the dog has developed primary seborrhea in the last 6 months and prior to that had no history of skin disease. She is seeking a second opinion because the dog's scaling is nonresponsive to topical antiseborrheic shampoo therapy. The 'sudden' development of primary seborrhea in a middle-aged dog with no prior history of skin disease seems suspect. The owner does not practice flea control. The dog is professionally groomed every 4 weeks. Flea combings reveal large amounts of dander, but microscopic examination of the debris does not reveal any organisms. Skin scrapings of a scaly area reveal numerous thick-walled organisms (120b). These are parasite eggs.
i. What is the parasite?
ii. What species of this parasite is most likely found on dogs?
iii. This condition is considered a zoonosis. Can the parasite reproduce on humans?

121 A 5-year-old dog was normal until 6 months ago when the owner started noticing that the dog's hair coat was changing color (121). The dog is nonpruritic and has no history of trauma to the area. Lesions are limited to the dog's head. No other skin lesions are found on the dog.
i. What is the general term for the clinical condition shown, what are the possible causes, and, what are the treatment options?
ii. What is vitiligo?
iii. What is tyrosinase, and what clinical disorder has been associated with its deficiency?

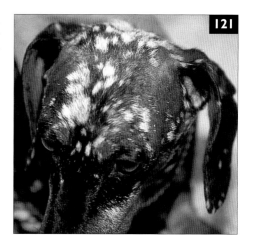

120, 121: Answers

120 i. *Cheyletiella.* *Cheyletiella* mite is a highly contagious parasite that affects dogs, cats, rabbits, and ferrets. The primary distribution of lesions is dorsal, and the classic history is a dog with little or no pruritus to moderate pruritus and scaling. It is a common parasite in dogs that require frequent grooming. This dog's primary idiopathic seborrhea resolved after the dog was treated for cheyletiellosis. Interestingly, the owners did not consider the dog pruritic.
ii. *C. yasguri* is most commonly isolated from dogs while *C. blakei* and *C. parasitovorax* are isolated more commonly from both cats and dogs.
iii. This mite has not been shown to multiply on people, which is in contrast to what has been found with respect to *Sarcoptes scabiei* mites.

121 i. Depigmentation or hypopigmentation. This can be caused by genetic disorders, breed associated diseases, or it can be acquired. Leukotrichia is the term used to describe depigmentation of the hairs, and leukoderma is the term used to describe depigmentation of the skin. This is a case of acquired hypopigmentation; the dog was born with normal coat color. The possible causes of hypopigmentation of the skin and/or hair include inflammation, drugs, metabolic diseases, neoplasia, immune-mediated diseases, and idiopathic. In most cases the cause is unknown. Post-inflammatory hypopigmenation is seen commonly in the inguinal region at healing sites of bacterial pyoderma.
Subcutaneous and topical glucocorticoids are notorious for causing depigmentation. Metabolic causes are rarely documented but include zinc, copper, and lysine deficiencies. Depigmentation of the nose, gums, and oral mucosa can occur in dogs with cutaneous lymphoma (pategoid reticulosis). Cutaneous lupus erythematosus and uveodermatologic syndrome are two well-recognized autoimmune skin diseases that can cause depigmentation of the mucous membranes. If there is an identifiable underlying cause that can be treated, the skin and/or hair may repigment; otherwise, there are no specific treatments.
ii. Vitiligo is another term used to describe depigmentation. The cause of vitiligo is unknown; however, there appears to be a genetic predisposition for depigmentation, and the cause may be immune-mediated. Leukotrichia and leukoderma are often used interchangeably with the term 'vitiligo', but this is best avoided unless there is a clear diagnosis of a genetic and/or immune-mediated etiology.
iii. Tyrosinase is an enzyme that is needed to produce melanin. Documented deficiency of this enzyme was found in chow chow puppies (Scott, 2001j). Their normally blue-black tongue turned pink, the hair coat shafts turned white, and there was rapid depigmentation of the oral mucosa. There is no treatment, and the disease is diagnosed by skin biopsy. Suspect specimens are incubated with tyrosinase, and melanin is found using special stains. Spontaneous resolution of the condition may occur.

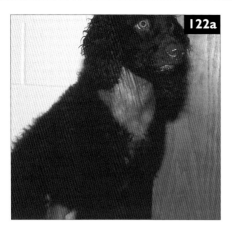
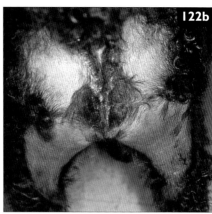

122 The neck, caudal thigh, and perineal region of a 1-year-old female Portuguese water dog is shown (122a, b). The hair loss began at approximately 6 months of age and has progressed. The dog is nonpruritic. Skin biopsy reveals a decrease in number and size of the hair follicles and hair bulbs.
i. What is the cause of this dog's hair loss, and how is this condition treated?
ii. What is a tardive alopecia?

123 The abdomen of an 8-year-old female cat is shown (123). The cat was originally presented for a cat bite abscess in this area. The abscess was surgically drained, flushed, and the cat was treated with 10 days of oral amoxicillin. Over the last 4 months, the surgical drainage site has failed to heal. The site opens and drains a blood-tinged fluid. Repeated surgery to remove granulation tissue and close the wound has failed to resolve the problem.

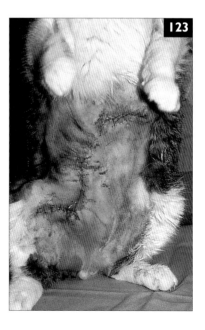

i. What is this cat's 'dermatological problem' and what differential diagnoses should be considered?
ii. What diagnostic tests are indicated? What is a Ziehl-Neelsen stain?
iii. What are Runyon group IV bacteria?

122 i. This is a case of pattern baldness of Portuguese water dogs. Affected dogs are born with a normal hair coat, and as they age, they develop a well-demarcated regional hair loss pattern. This syndrome is also seen in American water spaniel dogs. This is a hereditary disorder and affected individuals should not be bred from. Dog breeders are well aware of this skin disease and are not breeding from affected dogs, greatly decreasing the frequency of this condition. There is no known treatment, but some dogs respond to oral melatonin (3–6 mg q8h) or subcutaneous melatonin implants (1–3 × 12 mg implants). If treatment is efficacious, hair growth should be seen within 45–60 days.

ii. In tardive alopecia, the animal is born with a normal hair coat, and as the animal matures, focal, regional, or generalized hair loss occurs.

123 i. Nonhealing wound. The differential diagnoses include foreign body, immunosuppression, subcutaneous mycoses, sterile panniculitis, and infectious agents (atypical mycobacterial infections, *Nocardia*, *Yersinia pestis*, L-form bacteria).

ii. The cat should be tested for FeLV and FIV. The area should be radiographed for evidence of a foreign body and surgically explored. Finally, tissue biopsies should be collected for histopathology and bacterial and fungal culture. It is important to obtain large deep wedge sections for biopsy and culture. Many of the organisms in the differential diagnosis list, particularly atypical mycobacteria, are present in small numbers and/or are found in or near the subcutaneous fat. Furthermore, it is important to tell the laboratory processing the cultures and skin biopsy specimens which organisms are suspected as this will influence the choice of culture media and tissue stains, respectively. Because of the difficulty in isolating many of these infectious agents, impression smears of cut sections of tissue should be made and submitted unstained with the biopsy specimen. Cut sections of the tissue are blotted on a paper towel until 'dry' (i.e. all blood is removed) and then 10–12 imprints on clean glass slides are made. This cat had an atypical mycobacterial infection.

A rapid Ziehl–Neelsen stain is an acid-fast stain used to identify organisms such as atypical mycobacteria (e.g. *Mycobacterium fortuitum*, *M. chelonei*). Alcohol processing used in paraffin embedding can cause acid-fast organism to stain poorly.

iii. Runyon group IV mycobacteria include organisms such as *M. fortuitum*, *M. chelonei*, *M. phei*, *M. segmatis*. These are considered 'atypical mycobacteria' because they are rapidly growing unlike other mycobacterial organisms. These organisms are Gram-positive, acid-fast, aerobic, nonspore-forming bacilli. They are ubiquitous in nature. The slow growing mycobacteria are rarely associated with primary skin lesions; skin lesions are usually secondary to systemic involvement.

124 A 4-year-old female spayed St. Bernard dog is presented for the problem of facial odor and recurrent facial 'hot spots'. The dog has no other dermatological problems. According to the owner, the dog developed a facial hot spot 1 year ago, and the lesion never resolved. It responds to glucocorticoid therapy, but always returns. The lesion is very painful and malodorous. Upon physical examination it is noted

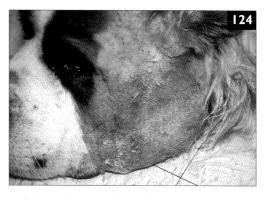

that almost the entire lateral aspect of the right side of the dog's face is involved (**124**). The skin is hot, moist, exudative, and edematous. There is a serous crust attached to the hairs and, at the margin of the lesion, a papular eruption is visible. An examination of the dog's oral cavity and ears is performed to look for a cause of the unilateral lesion and none is found. A review of the patient's medical record reveals the lesion has been consistently skin scraping negative. Impression smears of the lesion today, and in the past, have shown neutrophilic inflammation with intercellular and extracellular cocci. The lesion was treated with topical chlorhexidine scrubs and prednisone (0.5 mg/kg for 5–10 days). The dog had received one course of oral antibiotic therapy (amoxicillin 500 mg q12h for 10 days).
i. What are the possible reasons for failure of this lesion to resolve?
ii. What treatment recommendations should be made?

125 The medial pinna of a severely atopic West Highland white terrier dog is shown (**125**). Both of the dog's ears appear similar. Note the severe erythema, lichenification, and scaling. The owners arrived home to find the dog with its head tilted to the left side and a soft fluctuant bulging on the medial aspect of the left ear pinna.

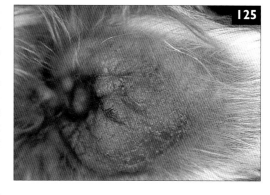

i. What is the most likely diagnosis?
ii. The owners don't believe the diagnosis. How can it be confirmed?
iii. What is the most likely cause of this condition, and what are the treatment options?

124 i. First, this is primarily a bacterial skin disease and glucocorticoid therapy is inappropriate. Second, the antimicrobials therapy prescribed was ineffective for a number of reasons. The dosage for this patient was too low and the length of therapy too short. Third, amoxicillin is a poor empirical choice of antibiotics for treatment of *Staphylococcus intermedius*. Finally, it is very possible that there is an underlying skin disease perpetuating the lesions. Recurrent areas of pyotraumatic dermatitis on the face are common in atopic dogs.

ii. The first treatment step has already been done, clipping of the hair coat from the lesions. Next, the area should be washed gently with an antibacterial shampoo or scrub. The owner can continue to do this at home on a daily basis provided the dog does not object. Finally, the lesion should be treated with systemic antibiotics (e.g. cephalexin 30 mg/kg PO q12h) for at least 4–6 weeks. This is a very large dog and the owner must understand the dog must be dosed based upon the dog's weight. If the lesion recurs after appropriate therapy, a more aggressive search for an underlying cause or trigger should be pursued. At this time, it is uncertain if the relapses are due to the presence of an underlying trigger or solely due to treatment errors.

125 i. Aural hematoma.

ii. The diagnosis can be confirmed by aspirating fluid (i.e. blood) from the swelling. This should be done with a small gauge needle because it is painful, and the pressure within the hematoma will cause it to ooze blood.

iii. Aural hematomas are caused by violent head shaking that fractures the cartilage, leading to hemorrhage within the delicate ear cartilage. Clinically, this appears as a soft fluctuant swelling on the concave surface of the pinnae. Unilateral or bilateral aural hematomas are common in atopic dogs; many atopic dogs have curled or deformed ear pinnae suggesting they have had previous aural hematomas that were untreated and allowed to self-heal. The most common cause of aural hematomas in cats is an ear mite infestation.

Aural hematomas, although uncomfortable for the patient, are not life threatening and will resolve without treatment in most cases but with scarring. Optimum repair of an aural hematoma requires surgical drainage of the lesion and closure of the dead space with sutures. The two most common mistakes made when repairing aural hematomas are use of too few sutures (i.e. leaving too much dead space) and removing the sutures before the ear has completely healed (i.e. >3 weeks). Mastitis teat cannulas can be used for temporary relief of the swelling, or in patients that cannot tolerate general anesthesia. This is an excellent temporary measure for dogs presented for an emergency examination. Laser therapy is an option to cold surgery and sutures; however, the cosmetic success of either procedure depends more upon the skill of the surgeon than on the tool.

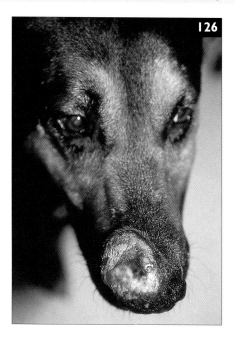

126 In a stray animal shelter, one of the volunteers identifies a dog with 'nasal fungus'. Examination of the dog (126) reveals a raised, destructive, proliferative lesion involving the left naris and soft tissue of the nose. The area is necrotic and malodorous, and the dog's regional lymph nodes are enlarged. The major question the volunteer needs answered is whether or not the dog can be treated and made available for adoption.

i. What are the differential diagnoses, and what diagnostic tests are indicated at this time?

ii. What prognostic factors need to be assessed in dogs with canine MCT?

iii. What is the significance of each of these prognostic factors?

127 What is feline paraneoplastic alopecia?

126, 127: Answers

126 i. The most likely cause is a tumor: MCT, fibrosarcoma, melanoma, and carcinoma. Other causes include bacterial or fungal granuloma, kerion reaction, subcutaneous mycoses, and trauma. The lack of history in this case complicates the situation because there is no knowledge of how slowly or quickly the lesion developed. Rapid development of the lesion does not preclude a tumor but is more commonly associated with infectious agents. In this patient, as in other cases, the most important question to answer is 'what is it?' From that perspective, FNA and skin biopsies are the most cost effective diagnostic tools. Once a diagnosis has been made, the owners can determine whether to pursue treatment or not. If treatment is pursued, additional diagnostics (e.g. skull radiographs) are indicated to determine invasiveness of the mass and treatment options. Diagnostics in this case revealed that this was an invasive MCT.
ii. The prognostic factors that need to be assessed include: histological grade, clinical stage, location, AgNOR count, growth rate, PCNA assessment, DNA ploidy, recurrence, systemic signs, age, breed, and sex (Thamm and Vail, 2001).
iii. Histological grade: this is strongly predictive of the outcome. Dogs with undifferentiated tumors usually die of the disease after local therapies, as compared with dogs with well-differentiated tumors that are usually cured with appropriate therapy. Clinical stage: states that are confined to the skin without local lymph node or distant metastasis have a better prognosis than higher stage diseases. Location: visceral or bone marrow MCTs have a grave prognosis. Tumors of the oral, mucocutaneous, perianal, preputial, and nail bed sites tend to be undifferentiated and are associated with a poor prognosis. AgNOR count: the AgNOR count is predictive of surgical outcome. The higher the AgNOR count, the poorer the prognosis. Growth rate: MCTs that remain localized for long periods of time are usually benign. PCNA assessment: immunohistochemical assessment of PCNA is a measure of tumor proliferation; the higher the score the more guarded the prognosis. DNA ploidy: aneuploid tumors are associated with higher clinical stage scores and shorter survival times. Recurrence: tumors that recur at the site of surgical excision carry a more guarded prognosis. Systemic signs: animals that present with systemic signs of illness (anorexia, vomiting, gastrointestinal ulceration, melena) usually have more aggressive forms of MCT. Age: older dogs have shorter median disease-free interval than younger dogs. Breed: MCTs in boxer dogs tend to be more differentiated and carry a better prognosis. Sex: male dogs tend to have a shorter survival time than female dogs post-chemotherapy (Thamm and Vail, 2001).

127 Feline paraneoplastic alopecia is a dermatological manifestation of a systemic disease, in particular neoplasia of the gastrointestinal tract. The most common presentation is an older cat presented with hair loss on the ventral abdomen and/or on the extremities. The footpads may appear thin and scaly. Sometimes there is a shiny appearance to the alopecic skin. Abdominal neoplasia should be suspected in any older cat presenting with a recent (weeks to months) history of overgrooming or hair loss.

128 A 9-month-old indoor cat was presented for a wound on the lateral thorax and matting of the hair coat. The owner reported that the wound started as a small swelling that gradually enlarged over the last week (128a). The kitten was not febrile, and the wound was cool and nonpainful upon palpation. The wound

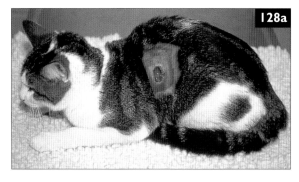

was explored, and a moving object was seen in the hole. A foreign object was removed from the wound (128b).

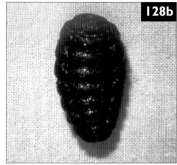

i. What is the object?
ii. How is this infestation treated?
iii. How did this kitten contract this parasite, and what is the primary host?

129 Coalescing erythema on the testicular skin of a dog is shown (129). The lesions blanche when a glass slide is pressed over them. Similar lesions are present throughout the coat of this dog. In addition, the dog was depressed and 'walking stiffly', according to the owner. These lesions were not present 3 days ago when the dog received his yearly physical examination, heartworm test, and appropriate vaccinations. At the

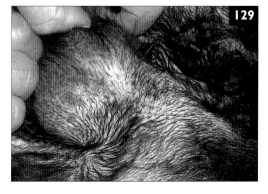

time of vaccination a bacterial pyoderma was found, and a 3 week course of oral antibiotics was prescribed.
i. What are the differential diagnoses?
ii. How should this case be managed?

128 i. *Cuterebra* fly larvae.
ii. Treatment is unnecessary since cats are not natural hosts for this parasite. However, the larva should be carefully removed. The wound should be enlarged enough to allow for the entire grub to be removed without breaking it: retained parts can cause infection, foreign body reactions, irritant reactions and, in rare cases, allergic reactions. The wound should be flushed after removal of the parasite, and a 7–10 day course of antibiotic therapy may be needed depending upon the extent of the secondary infection.
iii. *Cuterebra* are large bee-like flies that do not bite or feed. They lay their eggs on stones, vegetation, or near the openings of animal burrows. The natural hosts of this organism are rabbits and rodents. Cats and dogs become infested when they come into contact with the larvae on rocks, vegetation, or near the openings of rabbit and rodent dens. The larvae enter the body when ingested or via natural openings. The larvae undergo aberrant migration and localize to the skin of the neck, head, and trunk. *Cuterebra* infestations are seen most commonly in the late summer and fall. Lesions can be slow or rapid in development. Although *Cuterebra* infestations are most common in outdoor cats, they can be seen in housecats with no known outdoor exposure. This exposure occurred somewhere and sometime without the owner's knowledge.

129 i. The lesion depicted is a diffuse reddening on the skin of the scrotum. Potential differential diagnoses include: allergic or irritant contact dermatitis, worsening of the bacterial pyoderma, hemorrhage, and drug reaction.
ii. Because lesions are present throughout the hair coat, it is unlikely this is a contact dermatitis. However, the owners should be asked if they have washed the dog in the last 72 hours, applied any type of conditioner, and/or if the dog has been exposed to any unusual chemicals (e.g. lawn fertilizer). Impression smears should be taken to determine if the bacterial pyoderma has worsened, or if a concurrent yeast infection has developed. The blanching upon pressure is most compatible with erythema due to inflammation. If the lesion did not blanche, cutaneous hemorrhage would be included in the problem list. The most likely cause of the lesions is a drug reaction to the oral antibiotic prescribed for bacterial pyoderma. If this is a drug reaction, the lesions should resolve within a few days after halting administration of the drug. The lesions in this dog resolved within 72 hours after discontinuation of cephalexin.

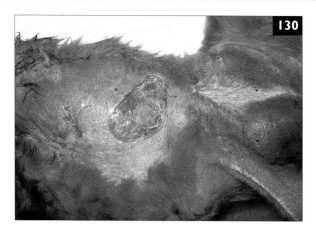

130 The abdomen of a 10-year-old Irish setter dog is shown. The owners presented the dog for a very large, subcutaneous, ulcerative mass in the caudal abdominal area (130). The mass was diagnosed via skin biopsy as a hemangiosarcoma.
i. What is the treatment of choice?
ii. What is the prognosis for this patient?

131 The PCR method is sensitive enough to detect as little as one DNA molecule in almost any type of sample, allowing scientists to investigate changes at the level of the single cell. Because PCR is such an accurate and sensitive diagnostic tool, it may soon be clinically useful for early detection or residual detection of disease. As an example, PCR was recently used for early detection of opportunistic and pathogenic fungi in dermal specimens from dermatomycoses-affected patients (Turin *et al.*, 2000), where early detection of fungal infection is essential for effective therapy. PCR may also be clinically useful for detection of conditions such as CSD, a disease difficult to diagnose in animals due to the quiescent phases of the infecting microbe (Tapp *et al.*, 2001). Thus, PCR may soon be an alternative tool replacing conventional detection techniques.
i. How does the PCR method work?
ii. How would you examine the products of a PCR reaction?

130 i. Wide surgical excision.

ii. The prognosis depends upon the location of the lesion. Dermal tumors have a good prognosis if excised completely, since they have a low recurrence rate. Tumors in the subcutaneous tissue have a poor prognosis because they recur at the original site and have a high rate of metastasis.

131 i. For PCR to work, one must know at least part of the DNA sequence of the segment to be amplified. Two oligonucleotides (or primers) are synthesized, and each primer is complementary to a short sequence in one strand of the desired DNA sequence. The primer sequences should flank the sequence to be amplified. DNA is isolated from a sample, and the DNA is heated briefly (denaturing step) to denature it. The DNA is then cooled (annealing step) in the presence of an excess of the synthetic oligonucleotide primers. The cooling allows the primers to anneal to the complementary sites within the desired segment. A heat-stable DNA polymerase (*TaqI*) and four deoxynucleotide triphosphates are added, causing the primed segment to be amplified (amplification step). The denaturing, annealing, and amplification steps are then repeated through 25–35 cycles. This process takes only a few hours on an automated thermocycler, and the amplified DNA is abundant enough within the sample that it can be easily isolated and cloned.

ii. As the sequence of the primers used in the reaction is known and their locations on the gene sequence of interest, it is easy to determine the size of a PCR product. For example, primer 1 recognizes bases 10–22, while primer 2 recognizes bases 500–518. Thus the size of the PCR product of interest is 508 base pairs (bp).

In order to visualize the PCR product, the sample is mixed with a loading buffer (usually TAE or TBE) containing a dye. The sample is then loaded into a 'well' in an agarose gel. Depending on the size of the PCR products, the concentration of agarose varies from 0.8–1.5%. The gel is then placed in a gel box along with a buffer and a current applied. As DNA carries an overall negative charge, it will migrate towards the positive electrode; the agarose gel acts like a net or screen allowing small products to move quickly through the 'holes' in the gel, while larger products move more slowly. Thus smaller products will migrate faster towards the positive electrode and will move to the bottom of the gel, and larger products will move more slowly and will be found at the top of the gel. Once the gel run is completed, the PCR products can be viewed using an ultraviolet light box. EB, a fluorescent dye, is usually added to the gel or the gel buffer before the run, allowing the EB to bind to the DNA. When EB is exposed to ultraviolet light it fluoresces and the DNA appears as an orange band on the gel. The gel can then be photographed and the PCR products analyzed.

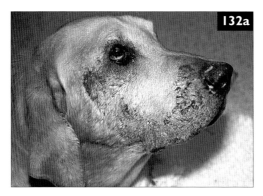

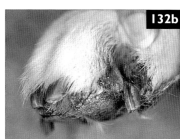

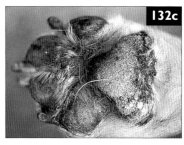

132 A 12-year-old mixed breed dog was presented for the complaint of lethargy, weight loss, polyuria, polydipsia, and skin lesions (**132a**). Dermatological examination revealed crusting, hair loss, and scaling on the distal extremities, especially on the elbows and hocks. Pedal hyperkeratosis, crusting and hair loss on the muzzle, and mucocutaneous ulcerations (**132b, c**) were also noted. Palpation of the abdomen revealed a small liver. Laboratory evaluation of the dog revealed a normochromic, normocytic, non-regenerative anemia, hyperglycemia, elevated serum alkaline phosphatase and alanine aminotransferase, and elevated post-prandial bile acid concentrations. Antinuclear antibody testing was negative.

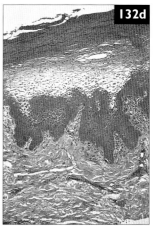

i. What differential diagnoses are ruled out based upon the diagnostic testing done so far?
ii. What differential diagnoses should be considered?
iii. Skin biopsy findings reveal the following: diffuse parakeratotic hyperkeratosis, upper level epidermal edema, vacuolation of keratinocytes, and epidermal hyperplasia. There is a mild superficial perivascular infiltrate in the superficial dermis. The pathologist comments that it shows the classic 'red, white, and blue' (**132d**) of 'X' disease. An ultrasound of the liver shows a 'honeycomb' pattern. What is the most likely diagnosis for the skin disease?

133 Endectocides are a new class of parasiticidal agents.
i. What are they derived from and what is their mechanism of action?
ii. What diseases are they used to treat?

132 i. The differential diagnoses that may be ruled out are PF, zinc-responsive skin disease, and generic dog food dermatitis. Dogs with these disorders rarely have laboratory abnormalities and/or the clinical signs described for this patient.

ii. Diagnoses that should be considered include systemic lupus erythematosus and hepatocutaneous syndrome (superficial necrolytic dermatitis, metabolic epidermal necrosis).

iii. The most likely diagnosis is hepatocutaneous syndrome. This is a cutaneous marker of systemic disease. Dogs with liver disease, chronic gastrointestinal disorders, glucagonoma, diabetes mellitus, and pancreatic tumors may develop this unique pattern of skin disease. The pathogenesis is unknown but is related to degeneration of the keratinocytes in the upper levels of the epidermis. The most likely cause is some type of nutritional imbalance caused by an underlying metabolic disorder.

There is no specific treatment for the skin lesions; however, supplementation with high quality protein (1 egg yolk/4.5 kg), zinc sulfate (10 mg/kg q24h), and fatty acids (e.g. omega-3 and omega-6 capsules) may be beneficial. Alternatively, infusions of amino acids (500 ml of a 10% solution) IV via a central catheter over 8–10 hours every 7–10 days may be helpful in some patients. If there is no response after 4–5 treatments, then it is unlikely the patient will improve with amino acid therapy. If there is resolution of clinical lesions, then the amino acid therapy is administered as needed. The author has observed some mild resolution of skin lesions in dogs where the underlying metabolic disorder was treated (e.g. diabetes mellitus). In most cases, however, the appearance of this skin disorder is associated with a severe disease, and most dogs die or are euthanized within 1 year of diagnosis.

133 i. These are parasiticidal agents that have activity against both external and internal parasites. They are derived from macrocyclic lactones produced by the fermentation of various actinomycetes. This drug class includes avermectins (ivermectin, doramectin, abamecin, selamectin) and milbemycins (milbemycin and moxidectin). These drugs work by partly potentiating the release and effects of GABA. GABA is a peripheral neurotransmitter in nematodes, arachnids, and insects. Avermectins and milbemycin are also agonists of glutamate-gated chloride channels. These drugs are relatively safe in mammals because GABA is limited to the mammalian central nervous system.

ii. These drug are most commonly used in veterinary dermatology for the treatment of *Sarcoptes*, *Otodectes*, *Demodex*, *Cheyletiella*, fur mites, lice, microfilaria, and nematodes. Drug doses and drug intervals vary for these diseases and not all of these uses are licensed and approved.

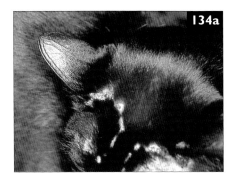

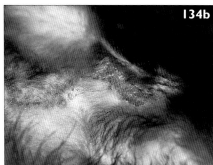

134 The owners of a 9-month-old Siamese–Burmese cross cat with nonhealing pruritic lesions presented the cat for a second opinion. The lesions were first noticed when the cat was 4 months of age. Physical examination was normal, except for the skin. Bilateral pinnal alopecia was present (134a) along with serpiginous lesions on the head.

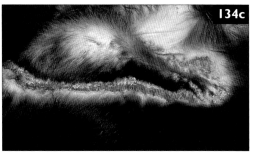

Erythematous linear lesions were present on the cat's lateral abdomen and in the inguinal region (134b, c). These areas were intensely pruritic and moist. The lesions were thickened upon palpation, but they did not feel like areas of linear eosinophilic granuloma. Previous diagnostics included skin scrapings, fungal cultures, flea combing, and a complete blood count. All test results were negative, and there was no response to flea control, a trial of ivermectin, a 12 week food trial, or antibiotic therapy. Skin scraping, flea combing, and fecal examination were negative at today's visit.

i. Impression smears of the lesions revealed eosinophils, mast cells, neutrophils, and cellular debris. What is the interpretation of this impression smear?

ii. Based upon testing to date, what differential diagnoses should be considered?

iii. What diagnostic tests are indicated at this point?

iv. The owners decline further diagnostic testing, but would like to treat the lesions symptomatically, if possible. What can be recommended?

135 Ivermectin is commonly used in veterinary dermatology for the treatment of various parasitic diseases. The oral and injectable formulations are available as 1% solutions. How would 10 ml of a 10 mg/ml concentration be compounded?

134 i. Eosinophilic exudation or inflammation.

ii. Previous diagnostic testing has ruled out parasitic causes of the pruritus and all commonly pruritic infectious skin diseases (bacteria, dermatophytosis). Today's impression smears did not reveal yeast organisms. The lack of response to flea control and a food trial makes FAD or food allergy respectively, unlikely. The likely differential diagnoses include atopic dermatitis, idiopathic eosinophilic dermatitis, and a histiocytic MCT.

iii. The two diagnostic tests that need to be done are skin biopsy to rule out feline MCT and intradermal skin testing and/or *in vitro* allergy test. Feline histiocytic MCTs tend to be characterized by multiple cutaneous nodules and serpiginous lesions.

iv. Ideally, a skin biopsy should be performed before prescribing symptomatic therapy. In this case, the most likely etiological cause is an allergic disease. This cat's lesions could be treated with oral or injectable glucocorticoid therapy. This patient's lesions resolved completely within 14 days of receiving a subcutaneous injection of methylprednisolone acetate (20 mg/cat). Eventually the cat was diagnosed as being atopic. This cat's primary allergens were to house dust mites. The young onset of clinical signs (approximately 4 months of age) is unusual.

135 This product is available as 10 mg/ml both orally and as an injectable form (Note: 1% injectable = 1 g/100 ml = 1000 mg/100 ml = 10 mg/ml).

In order to formulate 10 ml with a concentration of 1 mg/ml:
First, calculate the number of mg of ivermectin needed in the 10 ml solution:
  1 mg/ml × 10 ml = 10 mg

Next, calculate how many ml of ivermectin 10 mg/ml (stock 1% solution) is needed to get that amount:
  10 mg ÷ 10 mg/ml = 1 ml

Then, calculate the quantity of propylene glycol to add to get a 10 ml solution of ivermectin 10 mg/ml:
  10 ml – 1 ml = 9 ml of propylene glycol

Therefore, 1 ml of the stock solution should be diluted in 9 ml of propylene glycol to obtain 10 ml of a 1 mg/ml solution.

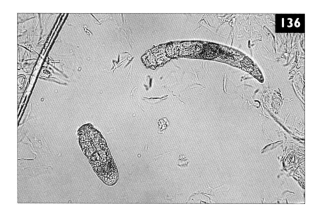

136 A 5-year-old Siamese cat was presented for the problem of psychogenic alopecia. According to the owner, the cat licks its abdomen furiously, bites, and growls when it grooms itself. The cat is an indoor cat. Previous skin scrapings, dermatophyte culture, skin biopsy, food trial, and blood allergy tests were negative or normal. The only abnormality noted was a mild eosinophilia on a complete blood count. The cat's pruritus did not respond to glucocorticoids. The ventral abdomen of the cat was 'painted' with mineral oil and wide skin scrapings over the area were done with a skin-scraping spatula. Mites were found on skin scraping after examination at 40× magnification (136).
i. What are they, and how are they treated?
ii. How do they relate to the psychogenic alopecia?
iii. Is this mite contagious?

137 What diagnostic test is shown (137)?

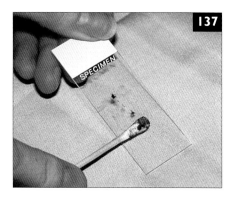

136 i. Feline *Demodex* mites. There is no licensed product for the treatment of demodicosis in cats. Otic demodicosis will often spontaneously resolve without treatment. However, preparations labeled as effective against ear mites will resolve infestations. Generalized demodicosis may occur in young cats and, in the author's experience, is very responsive to lime sulfur sponge-on dips once weekly until cured; cats often respond to therapy in 6–8 weeks. Alternatively, milbemycin oxime (2–3 mg/kg PO q24h) until cured is equally effective. The development of generalized demodicosis, especially in older cats, is often associated with an underlying systemic illness such as diabetes mellitus, hyperadrenocorticism (naturally occurring or iatrogenic), chronic renal failure, FIV, FeLV, or neoplasia.

ii. Feline demodicosis is an under-recognized cause of pruritus in cats. It should be considered in the differential diagnosis of any and all feline skin diseases associated with excessive grooming, e.g. psychogenic alopecia, atopy, food allergy, 'feline scabies', FAD, and contact dermatitis. These mites are easily overlooked and, if suspected but not found, cats should be treated with weekly lime sulfur dips for 4–6 weeks before more expensive diagnostics are undertaken and/or glucocorticoids are administered. In this case, the mites were found because wide areas were sampled via skin scraping, and the samples were examined under high magnification. These mites can be seen under lower magnification but are easily missed.

iii. Cats have three species of *Demodex* mites, but only one of them is contagious. The first is *Demodex cati*, and it is characterized by a long and slender appearance. It is most commonly associated with a pruritic dermatitis of the face, eyelids, periocular area, and neck. This mite can also cause generalized skin disease characterized by pruritus and hair loss. Generalized *D. cati* infestations are most often seen in older cats with underlying illnesses, e.g. diabetes mellitus. The second mite, *D. gatoi* is short with a blunted abdomen, and it is found in the superficial layers of the skin. This mite is believed to be contagious to other cats, unlike *D. cati*. It causes marked pruritus suggestive of 'feline scabies', atopy, or symmetrical alopecia and is easily missed on skin scrapings. The third species of *Demodex* mite, while unnamed, resembles *D. gatoi* but is slightly larger.

137 This illustration demonstrates how to prepare an ear swab cytology specimen. An ear swab from a patient is being rolled onto a clean glass microscope slide. It is important to remember that *Malassezia* organisms will stain poorly, if at all, if the slide is not heat fixed first. Heat fixing helps the organism to adhere to the slide and enhances staining. This is easily done by gently passing a lighter flame beneath the slide for 2–3 seconds. Excessive heating will damage the cytological specimen. Matches can be used but carbon may be deposited upon the slide during the process. *Malassezia* organisms are best identified under oil immersion.

138 The dorsal back of a 9-month-old Rhodesian ridgeback dog is shown (138). The dog was presented for the complaint of a nonhealing wound on the neck. The lesion has been present since the dog was a puppy. Impression smears showed neutrophilic exudate with bacteria, but the lesion did not respond to oral antibiotic therapy. On occasion, the owner reports the lesion drains a clear fluid. Exploration of the lesion reveals caseous debris and bits of what appear to be hair.

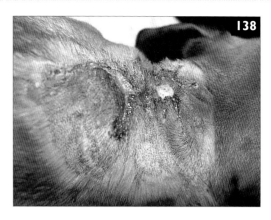

i. What is this lesion called?
ii. What clinical signs are associated with this condition, and how is this condition managed?
iii. How does the lesion form?

139 A 2-year-old springer spaniel dog was presented for the problem of odor and recurrent lip fold pyoderma (139). Systemic antibiotic therapy, daily facial washings, surgical lip fold resection, and a change of food bowls did not resolve the problem. The owner reported the dog rubbed his face after eating (normal behavior) and several times per hour on the floor and couch. The dog was currently eating a lamb-based restricted dog food.

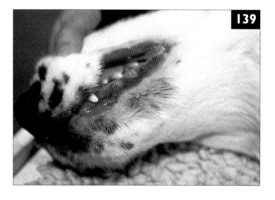

i. Standard interventions for lip fold pyoderma due to redundant lips (anatomical defect) have not resolved the problem. What other differential diagnoses should be considered?
ii. What initial diagnostic tests are indicated?
iii. What immunological mechanisms are believed to be responsible for the development of food allergy in dogs?

138 i. Dermoid sinus, a hereditary disorder of this breed.

ii. The clinical signs vary depending upon whether or not the sinus becomes cystic, inflamed, and/or if infection develops. In many dogs, the only symptom is a whirling of hair along the back with a palpable cord of tissue descending in the skin toward the spine. In some dogs, spinal fluid may drain from the lesion. If the sinus becomes cystic and filled with debris, the sac may become inflamed and infected. This appears as an area of pyogranulomatous dermatitis. Neurological signs may develop in infected lesions. No treatment may be needed if the sinus is not causing medical problems; however, cystic or infected lesions will require surgical removal although it is not always possible to remove the entire sinus. Meningitis is a possible complication of the surgery. Affected dogs should not be bred from.

iii. The dermoid sinus is caused by a neural tube defect. The sinus is caused by a tubular indentation of the skin from the dorsal midline to the subcutaneous tissue or to the dura mater of the spinal canal. The sinus ends in a blind sac, and the sac fills with keratin, sebum, debris, and hair.

139 i. The most obvious differential diagnoses are allergic skin disease: atopy and/or food allergy. It is also possible that the original diagnosis (redundant anatomical skin) was correct, but the continuing pruritus is due to an undiagnosed concurrent infection of bacteria and yeast (*Malassezia*). Finally, the regional anatomy should be carefully examined to make sure that the facial rubbing is not due to referred pain/discomfort such as otitis externa or dental disease.

ii. Cytological preparations of the lip fold exudates should be collected and examined for bacteria and yeast. *Malassezia* is commonly found in dogs with lip fold dermatitis, and it can cause intense facial pruritus. Skin scrapings for *Demodex* mites should also be done. If clinical signs compatible with pruritus are found, atopy and food allergy should be pursued. Skin scrapings were negative in this patient, and there were signs of pedal pruritus and otitis externa. The lip fold inflammation resolved with concurrent antibiotic and ketoconazole therapy, but the dog continued to lick its feet, roll on its back, and rub its face. Both intradermal skin testing and an *in vitro* allergy testing were negative. A diet trial with a different limited antigen protein (venison) was used, and the pruritus resolved but returned when the dog was fed a lamb-based diet. This was a case of severe *Malassezia* lip fold pyoderma secondary to a lamb food allergy.

iii. The immunological mechanisms involved in the development of food allergies in dogs are unknown. Based upon the clinical signs exhibited by animals shortly after exposure to an offending allergen, type 1 hypersensitivity reactions are well documented; however, type 3 and 4 reactions are also suspected to occur. Some animals exhibit clinical signs hours to days after exposure.

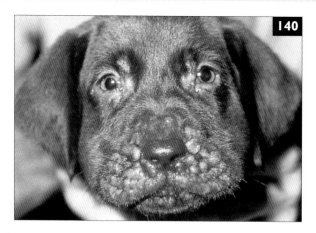

140 A chocolate Labrador retriever puppy was presented for the acute onset of facial swelling, depression, and anorexia (140). Upon physical examination, the puppy was found to be febrile and have generalized lymphadenopathy.
i. This is a classic presentation of what disease?
ii. What diagnostic tests are indicated, and what is the treatment of choice?
iii. What are the less common presentations of this disease?

141 A 3-year-old cat with a nonhealing lesion on its front paw is examined (141). The lesion was originally treated as a cat bite abscess several months before and it resolved, only to repeatedly recur. Today, the cat is febrile, depressed, lame, and has regional lymphadenopathy. Impression smears of exudate reveal acid-fast bacilli, repeated cultures are negative for bacterial growth, and biopsy reveals an epithelioid granuloma.

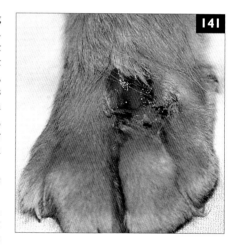

i. Which acid-fast bacteria are in the differential diagnosis?
ii. What is the most likely diagnosis, what are the treatment options, and what potential adverse reactions to treatment must be considered?
iii. Geographically, where is this disease most likely to be diagnosed?

140 i. Canine juvenile cellulitis or puppy strangles. This is an inflammatory granulomatous and pustular skin disease that affects the face, pinnae, and lymph nodes of puppies. The cause is unknown.

ii. The clinical signs can present as deep pyoderma or severe pustular dermatitis. The primary differential diagnoses are demodicosis, bacterial pyoderma, and drug reactions. Skin scrapings are needed to rule out demodicosis. Impression smears should be obtained to determine if there is a concurrent bacterial infection. Although not necessary for diagnosis, skin biopsy findings are consistent with granulomatous panniculitis. Glucocorticoids are the treatement of choice for this disease. Early and aggressive treatment is needed because this disease can be life threatening and can cause severe scarring. Prednisone or prednisolone (2 mg/kg PO q24h) is administered until the lesions resolve (10–21 days). After the lesions resolve, the dose of prednisone should be gradually decreased and tapered over a 30 day period. If glucocorticoids are discontinued too rapidly, relapse will occur. Topical therapy with warm antibacterial soaks may be used to remove debris and exudates.

iii. This disease can develop in older dogs (>6 months age) as periocular granulomatous dermatitis. Puppies may also develop nodular panniculitis alone or with classic lesions.

141 i. Feline leprosy (*Mycobacterium lepraemurium*) and atypical mycobacterium are both acid-fast bacilli. *Nocardia* spp. organisms are only partially acid-fast branching organisms.

ii. Feline leprosy, or *M. lepraemurium*, the causative agent of rat leprosy. The clinical signs are compatible with all of the considered differential diagnoses. However, the biopsy and cytological findings are most consistent with feline leprosy. In addition, the repeatedly negative bacterial cultures, even though organisms were seen on cytological examination of exudate, is typical of feline leprosy. This organism is very difficult to culture but can be identified via PCR from tissue specimens. Although lesions may spontaneously resolve, surgical excision is the treatment of choice for small well-circumscribed lesions. Some cats have responded to dapsone and clofazimine. Clofazimine is relatively well tolerated in cats with reddish-orange skin and adipose tissue being the major adverse effects. Dapsone, however, is more toxic to cats and can cause neurotoxicities, blood dyscrasias, and hepatic toxicity. Complete blood counts and serum chemistry panels should be monitored, and owners should be warned to alert the clinician if any neurological symptoms occur.

iii. Feline leprosy is most prevalent in colder wet climates such as the Pacific Northwest of the USA, Canada, New Zealand, the UK, and certain areas of Australia. Most cases occur in the winter (Noli, 2002).

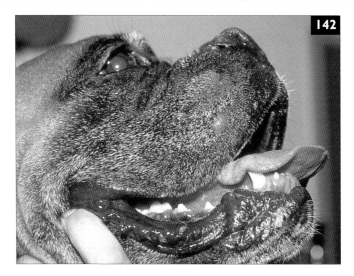

142 A 5-month-old male boxer dog was presented for evaluation of the small button-like mass on the lip (142). The owners of this dog have owned several other boxers, all of which died from one type of neoplasm or another. The owners are very agitated because this lesion developed very rapidly in their new puppy. The dog is otherwise healthy. Fine needle aspirate of the mass reveals sheets of round cells (histiocytes) with a high mitotic index.

i. What is the most likely diagnosis, what should the owners be told, and what is the treatment of choice?

ii. This disorder represents a spectrum of malignancies. Briefly describe them.

iii. What is leflunomide?

143 Where are *Candida* organisms found in the body?

142 i. Histiocytoma. This is *most likely* a benign tumor that will spontaneously regress and is common in all types of breeds.

ii. There are at least five histiocytic proliferative disorders of dogs. The most widely recognized is histiocytoma of young dogs. These are usually solitary lesions that spontaneously regress. Cutaneous histiocytosis is a benign skin disease that presents with multiple, erythematous, dermal to subcutaneous plaques or nodules. Lesions may be limited to the nasal planum giving the dog a 'clown nose' appearance. Lesions tend to wax and wane.

Systemic histiocytosis is most commonly seen in Bernese mountain dogs. It is a slowly progressive disease. Clinical signs include anorexia, weight loss, respiratory stertor, conjunctivitis, lesions involving the eyes, and multiple raised papules, plaques, and nodules over the entire body.

Malignant histiocytosis can be seen in any breed of dog, but the Bernese mountain dog is overrepresented and a mode of inheritance is suggested as a cause in this breed. It is usually a rapidly progressive and fatal disease with widespread distribution throughout the body, including skin, lymph node, liver, spleen, bone, bone marrow, and lung. Cutaneous lesions are uncommon, but are characterized by firm nodules in the dermis or subcutaneous tissues. Clinical signs include lethargy, weight loss, lymphadenopathy, hepatosplenomegaly, and pancytopenia.

Benign fibrous histiocytomas are rare tumors of dogs. These occur as single or multiple raised nodules on the face, legs, and scrotum. Malignant fibrous histiocytoma are rare malignant neoplasms, and they tend to occur in older dogs and cats. They are usually solitary, firm, poorly circumscribed, and have a tendency to be locally invasive to muscle and bone.

iii. Leflunomide is an immunomodulatory drug used in human medicine for the treatment of rheumatoid arthritis and in veterinary medicine for the treatment of hemolytic anemia and prevention of kidney transplant rejections. Recently, the drug has been used successfully to treat canine reactive histiocytosis (Cannon *et al.*, 2000). Cutaneous histiocytosis and systemic histiocytosis are also referred to as 'canine reactive histiocytosis'. The dogs responded to therapy (2–4 mg/kg) within 7–10 days. The most commonly observed adverse effects were vomiting, lymphopenia, and anemia. Glucocorticoids are often ineffective in canine reactive histiocytosis, and cyclosporin A, while expensive, offers an alternative therapy.

143 These organisms are normal inhabitants of the gastrointestinal and respiratory tracts and on the genital mucosa. In addition, it can be found in ears, nose, oral cavity, and anus of normal pets.

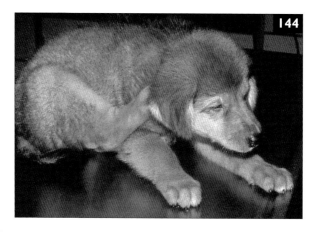

144 A newly acquired 12-week-old puppy was presented for severe pruritus. There was mild scaling present throughout the hair coat and a mild papular eruption on the ventral abdomen. When the earflap margin was rubbed an itch-scratch reflex was elicited (144).

i. What is the itch-scratch reflex associated with?

ii. The owner is very concerned about possible drug toxicity during the treatment of this disease. How should this concern be dealt with?

145 A 5-year-old male Labrador retriever dog was presented for examination. The owners were complaining about the lesions in the medial thigh and inguinal region of the dog (145).

i. What dermatological abnormality is depicted, what is the most likely cause, what other causes need to be considered, and what should the owner be asked?

ii. What diagnostic tests are indicated?

iii. How does this process normally occur in dog skin?

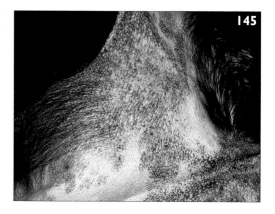

144 i. Severe pruritus associated with a papular eruption and a positive ear-flap test is most suggestive of scabies, but is not diagnostic. Other parasitic diseases to consider are demodicosis, fleas, and *Cheyletiella*; however, these parasitic infestations rarely cause severe pruritus. Impression smears, skin scrapings, and flea combings are indicated to rule out secondary bacterial, yeast, and other infestations, respectively.

ii. Concern over the possible toxic effects of antiparasiticidal drugs is reasonable when treating any pet, not just puppies. All effective antiparasiticidal drugs are associated with potential adverse effects and possible toxicities. Lime sulfur can cause oral and mucous membrane irritation and vomiting if ingested. Amitraz commonly causes sedation, pruritus, depression, polyuria, and polydipsia. Ivermectin can cause neurological signs such as tremors, salivation, sedation, seizures, and coma. In this case, skin scrapings were positive for *Sarcoptes* mites, and this puppy was treated with weekly lime sulfur sponge-on dips for 6 weeks.

145 i. Hyperpigmentation of the skin. This is commonly described as 'lacey hyperpigmentation' by veterinary dermatologists. The most common cause of hyperpigmentation of the skin is inflammation. Other causes of diffuse hyper-pigmentation include demodicosis, bacterial and/or yeast infections, endocrinopathies, alopecia X, flank alopecia, and ultraviolet light damage. In cats, dermatophytosis needs to be considered. The owner should be asked if this dog has any other clinical signs of skin disease. In particular, questions should focus on whether or not the dog is showing signs of pruritus. Atopic dermatitis is one of the most common causes of lacey hyperpigmentation in the axillary, inguinal, and medial thigh regions.

ii. Skin scrapings, impression smears of the skin, cytological examination of exudate scraped from within hair follicles, Wood's lamp, and dermatophyte culture (if suspected). Most importantly, a complete dermatological history is needed along with a dermatological examination. Although there is no specific treatment for hyperpigmentation, treatment of secondary infections and primary cause often results in a marked decrease in pigmentation.

iii. Melanin is produced in melanocytes, which are found in the basal layer of the epidermis and hair follicle. Melanin is formed within a melanosome, a specialized organelle within the melanocyte. Each melanocyte is associated with approximately 36 keratinocytes. Melanocytes eject melanin into keratinocytes via a process called cytocrinia. Skin color is determined by number, size, type, and distribution of melan-osomes. There are also dermal melanocytes but they do not transfer their melanin to cells. The exact mechanism of post-inflammatory hyperpigmentation is unknown.

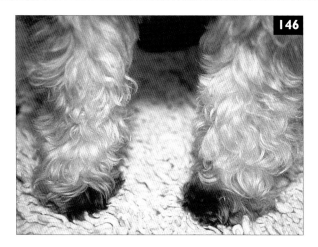

146 A 5-year-old schnauzer dog was presented for the problem of foot licking of 4 years' duration. According to the owner, the dog's activity was diagnosed as an anxiety related behavioral problem. Over the last 4 years, the owner tried various activity-related interventions, including hiring a dog walker and sending the dog to kennel to play every day. The dog walker and the kennel operator reported the dog chewed its feet regardless of the activities they offered the dog. The owner is seeking a second opinion because the problem is worsening and the dog's behavior is not altered by medications including mood modifying agents, tranquilizers, or glucocorticoids. Note the salivary staining on the feet (146).
i. What are the most common causes of foot licking in dogs?
ii. What diagnostic tests are indicated?
iii. What role might the *Malassezia* organism play in the development of clinical signs in this patient?

147 Amitraz is the active ingredient in the products Tactic® 12.5% (large animal formulation) and Mitaban® 19.9% (small animal formulation). Normally, 10.6 ml of Mitaban® is diluted in 2 gallons (9.2 litres) of water and then used as a sponge-on treatment. If the small animal formulation was unavailable how should the amount of Tactic® to use in place of the 10.6 ml Mitaban® be calculated?

146 i. The most common causes of pedal pruritus include: demodicosis, atopy, food allergy, contact allergy, bacterial or yeast infections, hookworm dermatitis (usually on the ventral aspect of feet), and behavioral causes.

ii. Material for a cytological examination should be collected before doing a skin scraping using mineral oil. Black/brown debris from beneath the nail, around nail, and/or between the interdigital webbing should be scraped off with a skin scraping spatula or scalpel blade and smeared onto a glass slide, heat fixed, and stained. Intense foot licking in dogs is a common clinical sign of *Malassezia* infections.

This is a case of *Malassezia* dermatitis due to atopy in a dog. The dog was treated with oral ketoconazole (5–10 mg/kg q24h) for 30 days and a topical antifungal shampoo, which resolved the pruritus. Alternatively, the owner could have washed the dog's feet daily for 5–10 minutes with an antifungal shampoo alone containing ketoconazole or miconazole. It has been the author's experience that topical therapy alone is less effective than systemic therapy with or without concurrent topical therapy. The dog was eventually diagnosed with seasonal atopy. The year round pruritus was due to a combination of seasonal atopy that triggered a secondary yeast infection that went undiagnosed.

iii. *Malassezia* organisms are part of the normal flora of the skin. They readily colonize the skin when the microenvironment favors their growth; in this case, increased humidity from licking may have been a key factor. There is evidence *Malassezia* contributes to the development of pruritus in atopic dogs via the production of antigens that cause a type 1 hypersensitivity reaction; concurrent infections may augment the pruritus. Dogs with atopic dermatitis and *Malassezia* dermatitis have significantly greater intradermal skin test reactions to *Malassezia* antigens than atopic dogs without *Malassezia* dermatitis. In addition, dogs with yeast infections have higher concentrations of serum IgE against *Malassezia* than nonatopic dogs (DeBoer and Marsella, 2001).

147 First, calculate the number of grams of amitraz needed for the Mitaban® dilution:

(19.9% = 19.9 g amitraz/100 ml of solution)
19.9 g amitraz/100 ml of solution × 10.6 ml of solution = 2.1 g amitraz

Then calculate how many ml of Tactic® is needed to get the same amount:

(12.5% = 12.5 g amitraz/100 ml of solution)
2.1 g amitraz ÷ 12.5 g of amitraz/100 ml of solution = 16.8 ml of Tactic®

Therefore, 16.8 ml of Tactic® can be used in the dilution in place of 10.6 ml of Mitaban®.

148 A 3-year-old male cat was presented for the lesion shown (148). The lesion reportedly developed rapidly, and it is unclear if the cat is pruritic or not.
i. What is the common name for the lesion depicted?
ii. What is the etiology? What diagnostics are indicated? How should the lesion be treated?
iii. What are the histological features of this condition?

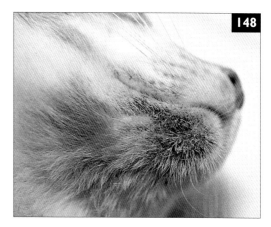

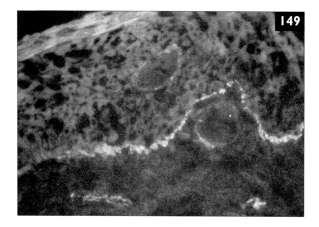

149 A photomicrograph of positive direct immunofluorescence testing from a skin biopsy of a dog is shown (149).
i. What pattern of immunofluorescence is shown?
ii. What common autoimmune skin diseases show this pattern?
iii. What diagnostic test will help differentiate epidermolysis bullosa acquisita from mucous membrane pemphigoid or BP?

148 i. Feline chin acne.

ii. Feline chin acne is not a 'diagnosis', but rather a clinical finding. The classic presentation is a primary disorder of keratinization. In these cats, there is marked comedone production on the chin and lower lip. Feline chin acne may also develop in some cats without a history of lesions as they age. These cats tend to develop scattered comedones that do not become problematic. Dermatophytosis, bacterial pyoderma, *Malassezia*, and demodicosis can trigger feline acne lesions very similar to those pictured. In some multi-cat households, feline acne can appear to be 'contagious'. These outbreaks have been associated with fungal or bacterial diseases, and in one case contagious demodicosis. Finally, atopic cats will rub their face and chin causing these lesions.

If the lesions are mild (just a few scattered comedones) the best approach may be to practice 'watchful neglect' and have the owner bring the cat back if the lesions spread. In cases like the one shown, material should be scraped off the chin using a skin-scraping spatula and smeared on a slide for cytological examination. A dermatophyte culture should be performed if the cat is newly acquired, goes outside, or is from a multi-cat household. Finally, skin scrapings for *Demodex* mites should be performed.

If the lesions are mild and there is no discomfort to the cat, no treatment is required. If the lesions are severe, the above diagnostics should help determine appropriate treatment. Bacterial infections should be treated for 21–30 days with antibiotics (e.g. cephalexin 30 mg/kg PO q12h) or longer if there is severe furunculosis. Yeast infections respond well to itraconazole (5–10 mg/kg PO q24h) for 21–30 days. These antimicrobials may need to be given concurrently. Topical therapy can vary from daily to every other day washings with a mild follicular flushing shampoo (e.g. benzoyl peroxide or combined antibacterial/antifungal shampoos), or antiseborrheic shampoo. Tar-based shampoos should be avoided in cats due to possible irritant or toxicity concerns. It is the author's experience that topical shampoo or ointment therapy, although often effective, fails due to lack of compliance by either the owner or the cat. Topical mupirocin ointment, topical glucocorticoids, or vitamin A cream may be indicated in refractory cases. It is important to determine if persistent lesions are associated with pruritus or not. If so, underlying pruritic diseases such as food allergy and atopy should be pursued. A diagnosis of 'idiopathic feline chin acne' is a diagnosis of exclusion.

iii. The most common findings are follicular keratosis and plugging, dilation of hair follicles and comedone formation and, in advanced cases, folliculitis, furunculosis, and pyogranulomatous dermatitis.

149 i. The pattern is positive basement membrane immunofluorescence staining.

ii. This pattern of immunofluorescence is most commonly associated with SLE, lupus erythematosus, BP, linear IgA bullous dermatosis, and epidermolysis bullosa acquisita.

iii. The diagnostic test needed is salt split substrates.

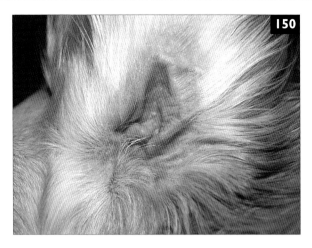

150 A 6-year-old golden retriever dog is presented in the winter for the complaint of bilateral otitis of 4 years' duration (150). The owners report that the dog's episodes are worse in the summer. The dog rubs and scratches at his ears and face and licks his paws. The owners clean the ears regularly often removing black waxy debris. Upon physical examination, the dog is otherwise healthy except for mild salivary staining of the paws, broken whiskers, and hair lodged between the teeth and gums. Otoscopic examination reveals bilateral erythematous otitis externa involving only the vertical ear canal. The skin of the external pinnae has a 'cobblestone' appearance. Cytological examination of exudates reveals mild ceruminous debris, squamous epithelial cells, and 6–10 *Malassezia* organisms per every high power field.
i. What is the clinical diagnosis?
ii. What is the most likely underlying cause?
iii. What treatment options can be offered to the owners for long-term management of this patient?

151 What are the most common side-effects of glucocorticoids?

150 i. This dog has otitis externa and a secondary yeast infection. *Malassezia* organisms are part of the normal flora of the ear canal but normally in numbers too small to be easily found. This organism should be considered a complicating factor when found on cytological preparations from patients with existing ear disease.

ii. There are two possible underlying causes of this patient's ear disease. First, it is possible that the underlying trigger or condition (e.g. swimming) that started the otitis is no longer present, and the dog's persistent ear infection is caused by an untreated secondary yeast infection. Second, it is possible that there is a persistent underlying skin disease causing the otitis and predisposing the dog to *Malassezia* infections. The history, breed, and other clinical signs (salivary staining of the paws, broken whiskers, hair lodged between the teeth and gums) suggest that he has an underlying pruritic disease. Atopic dermatitis (seasonal or nonseasonal) with or without food allergy is a likely cause of the otitis externa.

iii. At this point, it is important to determine if the dog's clinical signs are seasonal or year round. The most conservative approach would be to treat the yeast infection for 30 days and reevaluate the case. The author's preference is to treat with ketoconazole (5–10 mg/kg PO q24h) for 30 days and use a concurrent topical steroid-containing otic preparation once daily for 10–14 days. Other clinicians may elect to use aggressive topical therapy to treat the yeast otitis. The author uses topical therapy as a sole treatment approach in only select cases where a diagnosis has been made, and topical therapy is being used to contain symptoms, or when an episode is acute and less than 48 hours in duration. It is important to remember in this case that the problem has been ongoing for years, and systemic therapy is key to the diagnostic approach. The goal of treatment is to determine if the dog's otitis resolves, and whether or not the dog remains asymptomatic until summer. If the dog remains normal all winter but relapses in the summer, then the likely diagnosis is seasonal atopy (i.e. allergic otitis externa), and the most cost effective therapy would be medical management. If the dog's primary symptoms are allergic otitis, this patient could be managed with daily or every other day otic glucocorticoids during the months the dog is symptomatic. On the other hand, if the otitis externa resolves but recurs shortly after discontinuation of treatment and/or if the dog's ear disease resolves but he still rubs his face and licks his paws during the winter months, then the dog most likely has year round atopy and/or a food allergy. In this situation, intradermal skin testing and/or *in vitro* allergy testing and a food trial should be done to identify the allergens.

151 Polyphagia, polydipsia, polyuria, lethargy, panting, muscle wasting, exercise intolerance, secondary infections, slow hair regrowth, scaling, delayed wound healing, calcinocis cutis, and muscle wasting.

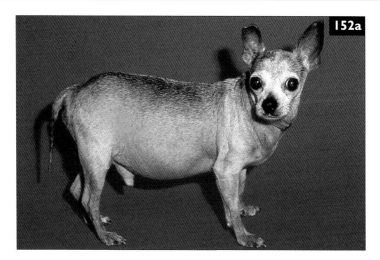

152 A dog was presented for weight gain, hair loss, polyuria, and polydipsia (152a). The owner is also concerned about the loss of the dog's ear tip. She reports the ear tip bleeds, becomes necrotic, heals, and then the cycle repeats. Physical examination of the ear tip revealed that approximately one-third of the right ear tip has been sloughed as a result of these cycles (152b).

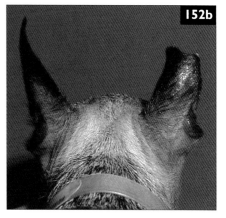

i. This dog is showing the classic clinical signs of which endocrine disorder?
ii. What are the possible pathophysiologies of ear tip necrosis in this dog?
iii. What other nonendocrine diseases can be characterized by ear tip necrosis?

153 The most common locations for cutaneous parasites to live are the superficial epidermis on the surface, attached to hairs and/or in the ears.
i. What are the most cost effective diagnostic tests for finding parasitic infestations?
ii. How are deep and superficial skin scrapings performed?

152 i. This dog is showing classis signs of canine hyperadrenocorticism. Note the bilaterally symmetrical hair loss, pendulous abdomen and prepuce, and 'rat tail'.

ii. Ear tip necrosis can be seen in cases of canine hyperadrenocorticism, particularly in breeds with small thin ear pinnae. The cause is unknown, but it may be related to micro thromboembolisms. Animals with hyperadrenocorticism bruise easily and the skin becomes thinner, possibly contributing to the development of these lesions. Finally, high concentrations of circulating glucocorticoids may affect healing of the lesions.

iii. Other causes of ear tip necrosis include vasculitis, lupus erythematosus, proliferative thrombovascular pinnal necrosis, cold agglutinin disease, feline auricular chondritis, and familial vasculopathy of the German shepherd dog. Feline auricular chondritis is characterized by swollen, erythematous ears that are usually curled and deformed. Familial vasculopathy has been reported in young German shepherd dogs. It is inherited via an autosomal recessive trait, and affected dogs develop alopecia, crusts, and ulceration of the ear tips. Depigmentation and crusting of the footpads may be seen along with lethargy and pyrexia (Ferguson, 2002).

153 i. Skin scrapings, flea combings, ear swab cytology, and acetate tape preparations.

ii. First a small amount of mineral oil is placed on the target area. Second, a fold of skin is pinched up and gently squeezed. Third, a scalpel blade or skin-scraping spatula held at 90° to the skin and gently used to scrape the skin until capillary bleeding is seen (**153**). Finally, the mixture of mineral oil and skin debris is scooped or

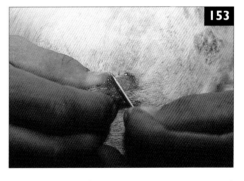

scraped off the skin and put on a glass microscope slide for examination. It is critical to squeeze the skin and scrape until capillary bleeding occurs when doing a deep skin scraping for *Demodex* mites; mites are found deep in the hair follicles, and this method optimizes their discovery. *Demodex* mites are part of the normal flora of dog and cat skin but in very small numbers. If easily found on a skin scraping of lesional skin, then their presence should be considered significant, and the patient has demodicosis. Superficial skin scrapings are done similarly except that the skin is not squeezed, and the scraping does not produce capillary bleeding.

154 A well-circumscribed mass on the lateral abdomen of a 5-year-old dog was aspirated (154a). The mass enlarged slightly after it was manipulated, and a MCT was suspected. FNA was performed, and the slide was stained with Dif-Quik. A photomicrograph of the aspirate is shown (154b).

i. What is the interpretation of the Dif-Quik slide?

ii. The photomicrograph (154c) shows cells in a blood smear from a dog. Are these cells of concern?

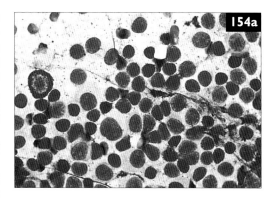

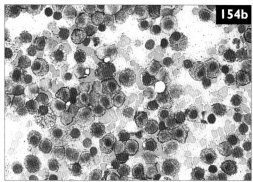

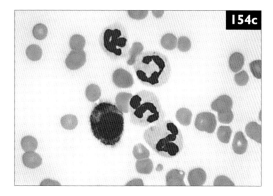

155 How should a superficial bacterial infection (i.e. impetigo) versus a deep bacterial infection be cultured?

154 i. This slide contains a uniform population of round cells. A MCT is suspected but distinct cytoplasmic granules are not clearly visible. A second slide was stained with a Giemsa stain, and the intracytoplasmic granules are much more clearly visible (**154b**). It is important to remember that the granules of less well-differentiated tumors do not stain well with Dif-Quik

ii. These are mast cells in the blood. These cells can be seen from time to time in normal dogs and do not necessarily warrant concern. In cats, mast cells seen in peripheral blood are always a concern and are usually associated with systemic mastocytosis.

155 Lesions for culture should not be surgically prepped or wiped with alcohol prior to sampling in superficial bacterial infections. An intact pustule is ruptured with a sterile 25 gauge needle (**155**), and a sterile cotton-tipped swab is used to collect the sample (blood and/or pus). Holding the swab at 90° (vertically) over the ruptured pustule and 'twirling' the swab while applying gently pressure is a common collection technique. Because there are *Staphylococcus* spp. on the clinician's skin, it is important NOT to touch the lesion.

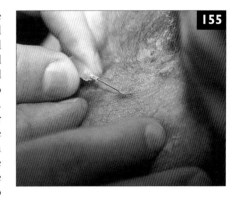

The techniques for culturing a deep pyoderma vary depending upon the presentation of the lesion. If there are intact furuncles present, samples can be collected as described for superficial bacterial infection or via aspiration with a sterile needle and syringe. In cases of severe exudation where there is contamination of the surface, matting of the hair coat, and/or a mixed population of bacteria seen on cytological smears is present, surgical prepping of the area is indicated. If there is a draining tract, a swab can then be inserted into the area. In cases where the infection is more diffuse, a deep wedge of tissue for culture should be collected using a scalpel and blade. Skin biopsy punches collect too superficial a sample; pathogens are often located in the deep dermis and/or panniculus. After collecting the sample, it is important to put it into sterile saline or transport media pending inoculation onto agar plates. In the case of tissue samples, the laboratory should be asked to macerate the tissue prior to culture.

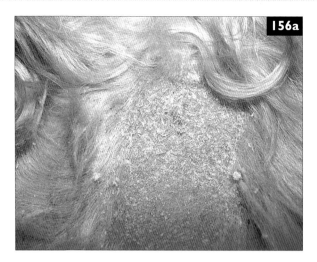

156 The skin of a 10-year-old female cocker spaniel dog presented for a second opinion is shown (156a). The owner's complaint is increasing generalized pruritus, excessive scaling, and diffuse erythema of 3 months' duration. The dog has no prior history of skin disease, and skin scrapings have been negative. There has been no response to flea control or ivermectin therapy. The dog did not respond to a 3 week course of oral antibiotics. Impression smears did not reveal any *Malassezia* organisms, and a fungal culture was negative. The pruritus is nonresponsive to glucocorticoids. Physical examination today reveals that the dog has generalized lymphadenopathy. Large sheets of exfoliating epidermal cells are present throughout the hair coat.
i. What diagnostic test is indicated and why?
ii. What is 'mycosis fungoides', and what is the current name for this disease?
iii. What are the clinical characteristics of Sézary syndrome or Sézary-like disease in dogs and cats?

157 What are the general functions of the skin?

156 i. A skin biopsy. It is important to determine what cell infiltrate is accounting for the diffuse erythema and scaling. Previous diagnostics have ruled out common causes of pruritus. The lack of a history of prior skin disease makes atopy unlikely, as does the lack of response to glucocorticoids. The age of onset of symptoms and the generalized lymphadenopathy are suggestive of a cutaneous lymphoma. On skin biopsy, histological

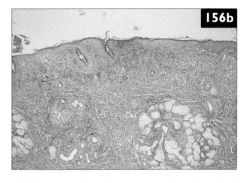

findings revealed that this dog had epitheliotropic lymphoma (previously called mycosis fungoides). One of the most common findings on a skin biopsy is a lichenoid (band-like) infiltrate beneath and into the epidermis (156b). The sudden development of generalized scaling, erythema, pruritus, and lymphadenopathy should raise suspicion. The prognosis for this neoplasia is grave.

ii. Mycosis fungoides refers to cutaneous lymphoma. The name originated from the human literature because the skin lesions associated with this disorder looked like 'fungi' growing on the skin. The current terminology is 'epitheliotrophic lymphoma,' a T-cell lymphoma that is difficult to treat. Treatments are considered palliative, and prednisone offers some relief from the pruritus. Cyclosporin A's antipruritic benefits have not been reported in dogs with cutaneous lymphoma. Retinoids have been reported to be effective in slowing the progression of the disease; isotretinoin (3–4 mg/kg q24h) is most commonly used. Drug combinations that have been most effective are those that include doxorubicin.

iii. Sézary syndrome or Sézary-like disease is subset of cutaneous lymphoma in dogs and cats characterized by the concurrent presence of cutaneous lymphoma and leukemia. Pruritus is common. The disease gets its name from the presence of circulating neoplastic lymphocytes with convoluted, hyperchromatic nuclei with a high nuclear:cytoplasmic ratio (i.e. the 'Sézary cell').

157 The general functions of the skin include: acts as an enclosing barrier or envelope for the internal organs, protects the body against the environment, produces adnexa (e.g. hair, claws, horny skin), regulates body temperature, storage (e.g. electrolytes, water, vitamins, fats), indicator functions (e.g. health, disease, physical identity, sexual identity), immunoregulation of the skin immune system, production of pigmentation for protection against ultraviolet light and for hair and skin, protection against infection, sensory perception, Vitamin D production, and secretion of sweat and sebum.

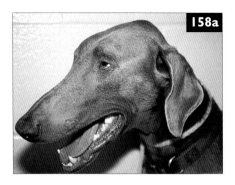

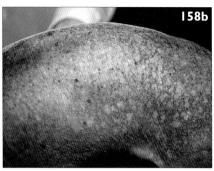

158 A 2-year-old blue doberman pinscher dog was referred for the problem of an 'endocrine alopecia' of unknown etiology. Previous diagnostic tests were normal or negative and included: skin scrapings, dermatophyte culture, complete blood count, urinalysis, serum chemistry panel, thyroid hormone evaluation, low-dose dexamethasone suppression test, and surgical neutering. Dermatological examination reveals a thin hair coat, nodular-like hair follicles, comedones, bacterial pyoderma, and scaling (158a, b). All of the other littermates are similarly affected.
i. What is the most likely diagnosis, and what is the cause?
ii. How is this disorder treated?
iii. What are the most common histological findings?

159 An adult mixed breed dog is presented for examination. The owners report the dog developed weeping lesions on his inguinal region. The inguinal region of the dog is shown. Note the diffuse ulceration and erosion of the skin (159). Similar lesions are present in the axillary region, oral mucosa, and at other mucocutaneous junctions. Intact vesicles are present on the soft palate. Except for the skin and a mild fever, the dog is otherwise healthy. There is no history of recent drug administration.

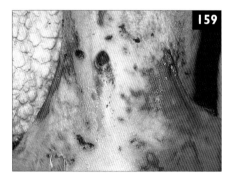

i. What are the differential diagnoses?
ii. The following histological findings were reported : subepidermal clefting and vesicle formation without acantholysis, DIF revealed a linear deposit of immuno-globulins, ANA testing was negative. The skin biopsy findings are incompatible with which of the differential diagnoses? What is the most likely diagnosis?
iii. How is this disease treated?

158 i. Color dilution alopecia (previously called color mutant alopecia). This is a genetic disorder of the hair coat commonly associated with a blue or fawn coat color. The cause is unknown, but it is believed to be due, in part, to a defect in the coat color genes at the D locus. Affected dogs are born with normal hair coats and, as they mature, they develop hair loss on the dorsum, recurrent bacterial infections, generalized thinning of the hair coat, secondary seborrhea, and cystic or dilated hair follicles. As hairs regrow, they grow more slowly and are often deformed. This disorder has been seen in cats with blue- or cream-colored coats.

ii There is no effective treatment for this disorder. In the early stages of the disorder, hair loss is caused by hair shaft fracture. As a result, excessive grooming and harsh shampoos should be avoided. It is important to control the recurrent bacterial pyodermas associated with this disorder. Affected dogs will continue to lose hair, and many are alopecic by 2–3 years of age.

iii. Common histological findings show melanin clumping in the epidermal and follicular basal cells, macromelanosomes in the hair shafts or hair bulbs, and follicular dysplasia. The melanin clumping and macromelanosomes are key findings for diagnosis of this disease.

159 i. The major differential diagnoses include SLE, BP, erythema multiforme, pemphigus vulgaris, drug reactions, candidiasis, and cutaneous lymphoma.

ii. The skin biopsy findings are inconsistent with candidiasis, cutaneous lymphoma, pemphigus vulgaris, and erythema multiforme. Lichenoid interface dermatitis is the most common histological pattern seen in lupus erythematosus. In this case, the ANA test was negative, and the dog was otherwise healthy. The histological findings and DIF are most compatible with BP or a drug reaction. However, the historical finding of no known recent drug administration make this unlikely. BP is a vesiculobullous, ulcerative, autoimmune skin disease of dogs and cats. It can affect the oral cavity, mucocutaneous junctions, and skin in any combination. There are several clinical presentations including the aggressive form described above. In addition, some animals develop lesions limited to the oral mucoca or footpads and nail beds. The disease is caused by autoantibodies directed against the BP antigen in the basement membrane resulting in clefting and vesicles in the skin and mucocutaneous regions. This was a case of BP.

iii. This disease is treated by a combination of immunosuppressive drugs such as prednisone or prednisolone, azathioprine, and chlorambucil. Treatment is usually life-long.

160 Raised, nodular lesions are shown (160) on the ventral aspect of a dog's paw. These lesions are painful, and the dog is lame. Ruptured lesions exude a blood-tinged, purulent exudate.

i. This is a common skin lesion, and it is often incorrectly referred to as 'inter-digital cysts'. This skin lesion is a common presentation of what type of skin disease and what is the correct term for this lesion?

ii. How is it treated?

iii. Skin biopsy may be needed to diagnose what parasitic disease that is often associated with recurrent pododermatitis?

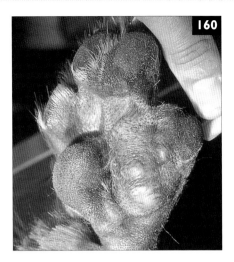

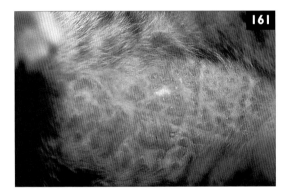

161 The caudal thorax of a 5-year-old cat is shown. Note the raised, erythematous plaque-like lesions (161). The lesions are exudative and intensely pruritic, and the owner reports the lesions are recurrent. Initially, the cat's lesions would resolve for 5–6 months at a time after treatment with methylprednisone acetate (20 mg/cat SC). However, over the last 2 years, the number of steroid injections required to resolve the lesions has increased, and the interval between relapses has shortened to 1–2 months. Skin scrapings, flea combings, and a dermatophyte culture were negative. Impression smears showed eosinophilic inflammation and exudation with no visible organisms.

i. What is the clinical diagnosis, and how should it be confirmed?

ii. What is the most likely cause of these recurrent lesions?

160, 161: Answers

160 i. These lesions represent deep pyoderma. Bacterial, fungal, neoplastic, inflammatory, and traumatic etiologies can all produce 'pyoderma' in the skin. The correct term for the lesions pictured is interdigital furuncle, and it should be noted the lesions are not 'interdigital cysts'. A true cyst is a non-neoplastic sac-like structure with an epithelial lining. Interdigital furuncles are common in dogs with pododermatitis. These lesions are painful, exude pus, and impression smears reveal neutrophils and bacteria. A furuncle is caused by an infection and subsequent rupture of a hair follicle. Interdigital furuncles may be single or multiple and are often recurrent. Scar tissue can often be palpated in the interdigital webbing where previous lesions have occurred. The misnomer 'interdigital cyst' is used because the lesions are fluctuant, recurrent, and rupture easily exuding a liquid-like material.
ii. The underlying causes of these lesions are multiple. Impression smears, bacterial cultures, and skin biopsy may be needed to determine/confirm the presence of a bacterial infection. If confirmed, the condition is treated with aggressive antibiotic therapy for at least 4–6 weeks (e.g. cephalexin 30 mg/kg PO q12h). Almost always, these lesions are the result of an underlying disease (e.g. atopy, demodicosis) predisposing the dog to pododermatitis. In some dogs, the lesions are the result of chronic friction, moisture, and maceration of the interdigital webbing leading to bacterial infection of hair follicles. Interdigital furunculosis is complicated by poor conformation, obesity, and foreign body reactions. Free hair shafts in the dermis, as a result of hair follicle rupture, create an inflammatory foreign body reaction that can result in chronic granulomatous inflammation perpetuating the lesions. In some cases, surgical excision or debridement may be needed to resolve the infection.
iii. Demodicosis. *Demodex* mites are often easily found on properly performed deep skin scrapings.

161 i. Feline eosinophilic plaques. Feline eosinophilic plaque is not a diagnosis but rather a dermatological reaction pattern that can be caused by parasitic, infectious, allergic, neoplastic, and idiopathic causes. This eosinophilic reaction pattern can be confirmed by skin biopsy. It is important to rule out proliferative (e.g. mastocytosis) or neoplastic skin diseases as quickly as possible to ensure proper therapy.
ii. Recurrent feline eosinophilic plaques are most often caused by hypersensitivity disorders such as FAD, food allergy, and/or atopy. Recurrent eosinophilic plaques and/or plaques that become refractory to previously effective therapies should make the clinician suspicious of allergic skin disease. Core diagnostic tests, including a trial of flea control, should be done before pursuing more expensive and time-consuming tests (i.e. food trials, intradermal skin testing, and/or *in vitro* allergy tests). This cat's lesions responded to monthly spot-on flea control; the cause of the lesions was flea infestation/FAD.

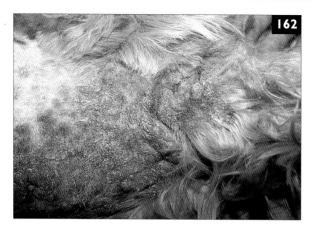

162 A 9-year-old male cocker spaniel dog with a life-long history of primary seborrhea was presented for examination of the ventral abdomen. The owner reported the dog developed the lesions slowly over the last month (162). The dog has gradually become pruritic, and the skin is malodorous. Dermatological examination reveals extensive hyperpigmentation, erythema, and crusting throughout the hair coat, most notable on the ventral abdomen. Individual hyperpigmented lesions have a waxy crust adhered to them and are bordered by erythema and a papular eruption. There is lichenification in the axillary region, and similar lesions are scattered throughout the dog's coat.
i. What is the working diagnosis? What in-house diagnostic testing should be performed?
ii. Assuming no complicating causes are found or pending laboratory test results, what treatments should be recommended?
iii. What are the most common ingredients in antiseborrheic shampoos, and which ones are most effective at removing scale?

163 Prior to the availability of commercially compounded enrofloxacin otic solutions, it was necessary to compound this preparation using the injectable formulation. How would 30 ml of enrofloxacin at 3 mg/ml be compounded? Enrofloxacin is available in a 22.7 mg/ml injectable solution.

162 i. Primary seborrhea complicated by secondary microbial infections (*Staphylococcus* spp. and/or *Malassezia* spp.). In-house diagnostic testing should include skin scrapings for *Demodex* or *Cheyletiella* mites, impression smears to confirm the presence or absence of yeast, and flea combings for mites and fleas.

ii. It is important that owners of dogs with primary seborrhea understand that the condition can only be managed and not cured. Attention to grooming details is critical. The hair coat is best kept at a very short length including the removal of any 'feathering'. This patient will require frequent bathing (at least 2–3 times a week) in medicated shampoos. The author would recommend alternating between an anti-microbial shampoo (single ingredient or combination product) and an antiseborrheic shampoo. In addition, antimicrobial therapy for at least 30 days will be needed. For example, if yeast were found cytologically, the author would treat this patient with cephalexin (30 mg/kg PO q12h) and ketoconazole (5–10 mg/kg PO q24h). It is the author's preference to treat both bacterial and yeast infections with systemic therapy especially if the dog is pruritic; concurrent therapy hastens resolution of pruritus. This patient had primary seborrhea and a dual microbial infection caused by bacteria and yeast. The lesions responded completely to a 30 day course of oral antibiotics and antifungal drugs, along with grooming and regular bathing. Subsequent relapses occurred if the owners became lax in the bathing routine.

iii. The most common ingredients in antiseborrheic shampoos are tar, sulfur, salicylic acid, benzoyl peroxide, and selenium disulfide. In an ultrasonographic biomicroscopic study of the ability of these ingredients to remove scale from the skin of dogs, selenium disulfide and colloidal oatmeal were the most effective, tar and sulfur-salicyclic acid were moderately effective, and benzoyl peroxide, ethyl lactate, and chlorhexidine were ineffective (Paterson *et al.*, 1999; Scott *et al.*, 2001d).

163 First, calculate the number of mg of enrofloxacin needed in 30 ml of 3 mg/ml solution:

3 mg/ml × 30 ml = 90 mg of enrofloxacin

Next, calculate how many ml of enrofloxacin at 22.7 mg/ml is needed to get that amount:

90 mg ÷ 22.7 mg/ml = 4 ml

Then, calculate the quantity of NaCl 0.9% to add to get 30 ml of enrofloxacin 3mg/ml:

30 ml – 4 ml = 26 ml of NaCl 0.9%

Therefore, 4 ml of the stock solution (22.7 mg/ml) of injectable enrofloxacin would be diluted in 26 ml of NaCl 0.9%.

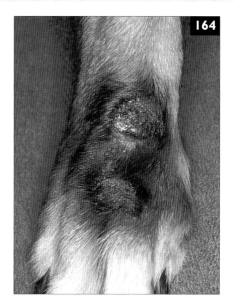

164 A 2-year-old dog was presented for evaluation of a mass on its forepaw (**164**). The lesion was raised, erythematous, moist, and firm to the touch. Closer examination revealed an erosive, circular lesion with a raised border; the lesion was slightly crater-like. A second healed lesion just distal to the first was also found, and extensive salivary staining was present on the paw. The owners reported the lesion had developed over the last several weeks, and this was the first occurrence of the lesion.
i. What is the clinical diagnosis?
ii. What are the two major causes of this syndrome? What core diagnostic tests need to be done at this time? What is the first line of therapy? How would treatment proceed if the initial therapy failed?
iii. What is a tail dock neuroma?

165 What is the difference between a pyrethrin and a pyrethroid?

164 i. Acral lick granuloma or dermatitis.

ii. The two major causes of this lesion are organic diseases and behavioral (obsessive–compulsive disorder). The latter is a diagnosis of exclusion, and this cannot be emphasized enough. Pruritus in dogs is manifested by licking, and in many dogs this may be the only clue that the dog is pruritic. Sometimes the differentiation between the two major causes is obvious. The dog has other compelling clinical signs of an underlying skin disease, there is a clear history of separation anxiety, or recent trauma/disruption in the dog's life. Clinical clues of an underlying pruritic skin disease may include signs of salivary staining on other limbs, a history of lesions developing on other legs in random fashion, and/or multiple lick granulomas occurring at the same time, or a history of trauma. Initial diagnostic tests should include skin scrapings to rule out *Demodex* mites, impression smears to look for bacteria and/or yeast, and dermatophyte culture to rule out mycotoic infections, especially if the lesion is acute.

Assuming the skin scraping is negative, and while the fungal culture is pending, oral antibiotics, e.g. cephalexin (30 mg/kg PO q12h) would be the first choice therapy. In the author's experience, more than 75% of these lesions respond to antimicrobial therapy. This indicates that this lesion has an underlying trigger, particularly if the lesion responds completely but recurs at a later time. Purely psychogenic lesions show only a minimal response to antibiotic therapy. The most common cause of recurrent acral lick granulomas is atopy; atopic dogs often have multiple lick granulomas on different limbs, and owners report that the lesions shift from one site to another. Lesions that do not respond to antimicrobial therapy should be biopsied to rule out foreign body reactions, kerion reactions, neoplasia, folliculitis, and/or furunculosis. Radiographs of the region should be taken looking for evidence of an underlying cause, e.g. fracture, osteosarcoma. The dog should be carefully examined for evidence of joint disease. Atopy and/or food allergies should be investigated before making a definitive diagnosis of psychogenic dermatitis.

iii. Tail dock neuroma is a rare complication of surgical tail docking. In this condition, the nerve endings regrow in a disorganized manner forming a neuroma. Clinically, this appears as a swelling at the tail tip that stimulates pain or some other unpleasant sensation causing the dog to lick, chew, or mutilate the tail. Surgical removal is the treatment of choice.

165 Pyrethrins are extracted from chrysanthemum plants and have immediate flea killing activity (fast knock down). They have little residual activity and are very sensitive to ultraviolet light. They are relatively nontoxic and are safe to use on young animals. Pyrethroids are synthetic drugs that are very stable in ultraviolet light. They work on sodium channels of insect nerve axons and cause nerve excitement and paralysis. They are rapidly adulticidal and have some repellant activity. Examples of pyrethroids include D-trans-allethrin, resmethrin, fenvalerate, and permethrin. Cats are especially sensitive to these drugs and they are best avoided in this species.

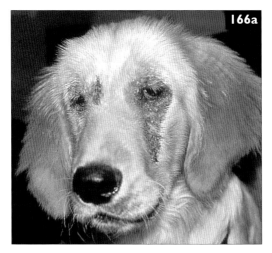

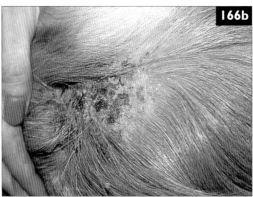

166 A 16-week-old golden retriever puppy is presented for matting, odor, and bleeding around the eyes (**166a**). The owner reported that the lesions began as focal areas of hair loss and rapidly progressed over the last week. Careful examination of the skin reveals similar lesions on the dorsum (**166b**). The areas are painful upon manipulation, but the puppy is otherwise normal. The lesions are erosive, exudative, and matted with serum and exudate. An impression smear of the lesions shows full fields of hypersegmented neutrophils, rare plasma cells, numerous macrophages, and red blood cells. Large numbers of cocci both intracellularly and extracellularly are also seen. A clinical diagnosis of deep pyoderma is made.
i. What is the most likely cause of deep pyoderma in a puppy?
ii. How should the puppy be treated?
iii. Recently, a zenograft mouse model has been used to study demodicosis. What are the highlights of that work?

166: Answer

166 i. Demodicosis. Rarely, deep pyoderma as a result of a kerion reaction may occur.
ii. If the puppy is febrile, it may require hospitalization and fluid therapy. After confirming the presence of the mite, oral antibiotic therapy for the deep pyoderma should be started and continued for at least 4–6 weeks. Impression smears should be done to determine if there is a mixed population of bacteria (rods and cocci) present. Topical therapy with amitraz at weekly intervals can be started once the areas of deep pyoderma are no longer eroded. This usually happens within 7–10 days. In this patient, whole body clipping of the hair coat and concurrent antibacterial shampoo therapy will speed resolution of the infection. Miticidal therapy should be continued until there are at least three negative skin scrapings at weekly intervals.

Alternative therapies such as daily ivermectin (600 µg/kg PO for at least 90 days) or daily milbemycin oxime (3 mg/kg PO for at least 90 days) can be used concurrently with the treatment of deep pyoderma. This is one indication for the use of systemic miticidal agents. Another indication may be a dog that is not tractable and/or cannot be treated topically due to owner related issues. The author treats dogs with demodicosis with weekly amitraz dips for at least 20 weeks before considering alternative therapies. If a progression from live to dead mites and immature to mature mites is seen, therapy should be continued. If not, then an alternative therapy should be considered. This puppy had generalized demodicosis that responded to weekly amitraz sponge-on dips.

iii. Recently, a zenograft mouse-model has been used to study the development of demodicosis. In this study, full thickness canine skin grafts from normal dogs were grafted onto SCID mice, and the canine skin was inoculated with *Demodex canis* mites. There were several interesting findings from this pilot study. First, large numbers of mites proliferated on the normal dog skin. If local immunity was the primary mechanism for controlling mite populations, this should not have been observed. This finding supports other studies that suggested that systemic host factors, rather than local immune factors, may be more important in the control of mite populations (Linder *et al.*, 2002). Furthermore, the study revealed that lymphocytes interact in a mechanism that may enhance, rather than limit, mite populations. Finally, mite proliferation did not result in hair loss unless secondary inflammation developed, contradicting a long-held belief that mites induce nonspecific histological changes in the skin.

167 A 12-year-old cat is pre-sented for weight loss, anorexia, depression, and excessive scaling (167a, b). The owner reports the cat developed these signs over the last 2 months. The cat has no previous history of skin disease and is not pruritic. The scales are large and thickly adherent to the skin. In addition, there is thick adherent debris in and around the nailbeds.

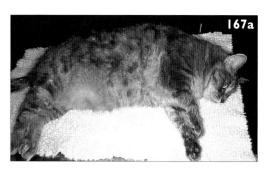

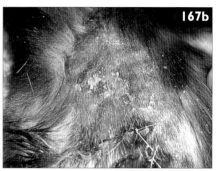

i. What primary differential diagnoses should be considered in this case?

ii. What diagnostic tests are indicated in this patient?

iii. Radiographs reveal a mediastinal mass. Histological examination of a skin biopsy reveals a cell-poor, hydropic interface dermatitis with large numbers of *Malassezia* organisms. What is the most likely diagnosis, and what is the prognosis?

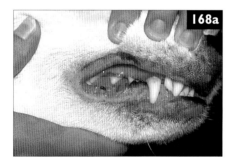

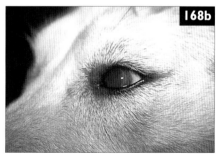

168 A 2-year-old male Siberian husky dog was presented for depigmentation of the lips (168a). Closer examination revealed he was photophobic and had areas of depigmentation on the margins of the eyelid (168b). The dog had difficulty navigating in the examination room, but the owner was not aware of any visual problems until the examination.

i. What is the most likely diagnosis?

ii. What would the dermatological and ophthalmic examinations be looking for?

iii. How should this disease be managed?

167 i. This cat has two major problems: signs of systemic illness, and exfoliative dermatitis. The major differential diagnoses for severe scaling in cats include pemphigus complex, generalized dermatophytosis secondary to an underlying disease, generalized *Malassezia* dermatitis secondary to an underlying systemic disease (e.g. FeLV, FIV), SLE, drug eruptions, cutaneous neoplasia, hyperthyroidism, and exfoliative dermatitis associated with thymoma. The age of the cat and the concurrent signs of systemic illness make it very unlikely this is a case of dermatophytosis alone; however, this should be considered because it can develop in cats debilitated from other illnesses.

ii. This cat will need both a dermatological evaluation and a medical evaluation. Skin scrapings, dermatophyte culture, impression smears of the skin and crusts, skin biopsy, a complete blood count, serum chemistry panel, FeLV and FIV tests, and radiographs of the chest and abdomen should be performed.

iii. The most likely diagnosis is exfoliative dermatitis and thymoma. Most thymomas are benign and surgical excision of the thymoma often results in resolution of clinical signs in cats. This was the case in this cat.

168 i. Canine uveodermatologic syndrome. This is a rare autoimmune disease involving the skin and the eyes. It is believed to be caused by autoantibodies against melanin, gangliosides, and photoreceptors. There is no age or sex predilection, but breeds such as akitas, chow chows, samoyeds, and Siberian huskies appear to be predisposed.

ii. The disease is characterized by depigmentation of the skin and acute concurrent uveitis. Depigmentation may occur on the nose, lips, eyelids, footpads, scrotum, prepuce, anus, and hard palate. The disease causes uveitis, photophobia, blepharo-spasms, lacrimation, injected conjunctiva, corneal edema, retinal detachment, cataracts, and glaucoma. If left untreated, these dogs may develop blindness.

iii. The skin lesions usually develop within 7–10 days of the ocular lesions; however, the owner is more likely to notice the depigmentation first. Because this disease can cause blindness, aggressive treatment and rapid diagnostics are indicated. Skin biopsies should be taken of the depigmented areas, and a thorough ocular examination performed. The eyes should be examined for uveitis. Life-long systemic gluco-corticoids and azathioprine will be needed to control the disease, and periodic ocular examinations should be performed to monitor uveitis. The skin lesions may respond to therapy but should not be used as an indicator of remission. Dogs may have active ocular lesions even though the skin lesions are static or have repigmented.

169 A 2-year-old cat was presented for acute, intensely pruritic, erythematous, exudative, raised lesions on the medial thigh (169a). The regional lymph nodes were enlarged, and skin scrapings and flea combings were negative. Cytological examination of an impression smear revealed predominantly eosinophilic inflammation (169b), and FNA of the regional lymph nodes revealed eosinophilic inflammation.

i. What is the clinical diagnosis?

ii. What are the most common underlying causes?

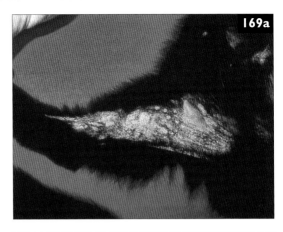

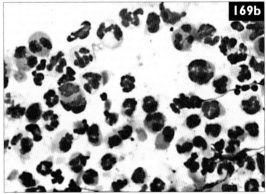

170 Ketoconazole, itraconazole, fluconazole, and terbinafine are systemic antifungal drugs used in veterinary dermatology. What are the mechanism, common adverse effects, and spectrum of activity of each drug?

169, 170: Answers

169 i. Eosinophilic plaque.

ii. These lesions were once thought of as a 'diagnosis', but it is now known that they represent a dermatological reaction pattern commonly associated with allergic skin diseases. The most common underlying cause is FAD. If lesions recurr or persist despite flea control, food allergy and atopy should be investigated.

170 i. Ketoconazole, itraconazole, and fluconazole are azole antibiotics. They work by inhibiting cytochrome P450 and the conversion of lanosterol to ergosterol, causing an accumulation of C14 methylated steroids. They also inhibit intracellular triglyceride and phospholipids biosynthesis, cell wall chitin synthesis, and oxidative and peroxidative enzymes. Side-effects and adverse effects are more common with ketoconazole than with itraconazole or fluconazole. Inappetence, vomiting, alopecia, and lightening of the hair coat have been reported as the most common side-effects of ketoconazole administration. Elevated liver enzymes are also common. Ketoconazole is embryotoxic and teratogenic. It can also suppress adrenal function.

Itraconazole is more potent than ketoconazole and can cause vomiting and anorexia. Adverse effects on adrenal function are not common with this drug. A rare vasculitis and necroulcerative skin eruption has also been reported in dogs. Hepatotoxicity can also occur with this drug and is most common in animals receiving high doses for long periods of time. When compared to ketoconazole, itraconazole is more potent. Fluconazole, when compared to ketoconazole, is more potent and is associated with decreased toxicity. Unlike other azoles, therapeutic concentrations are achieved in the cerebral spinal fluid. Fluconazole is the most fungal enzyme specific drug with respect to its mechanism of action, and side-effects are rare. High doses are embryotoxic and teratogenic; endocrine abnormalities are not associated with this drug.

The spectrum activity of ketoconazole includes yeast, some dermatophytes, *Candida*, *Malassezia*, and some of the dimorphic fungi associated with deep mycoses. Since the introduction of itraconazole and fluconazole, it is not commonly used as a 'core' therapy for deep mycoses as the other azoles have a better spectrum of activity. Itraconazole has a wider spectrum of activity than ketoconazole; it is more efficacious against *Microsporum* and *Trichophyton* than ketoconazole. In addition, it is efficacious against *Candida*, *Malassezia*, intermediate and deep mycoses (*Aspergillus*, *Sporothrix* spp.) and the protozoans *Leishmania* and *Trypanosoma*. Fluconazole has the widest spectrum of activity of the azoles, particularly against deep and intermediate mycoses.

Terbinafine is an allylamine that inhibits ergosterol biosynthesis and squalene epoxidase, which results in fungal cell wall ergosterol deficiency and the intracellular accumulation of squaline. This drug is both fungistatic and fungicidal. The major adverse effects are gastrointestinal. This drug does not affect cytochrome P450. This drug is used to treat dermatophytosis, sporotrichosis, candidiasis, and aspergillosis.

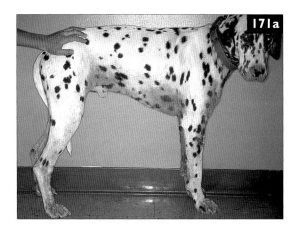

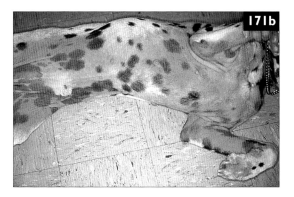

171 An 18-month-old male dalmatian dog was presented for the problem of intense pruritus (171a, b) in early June. The pruritus started when the dog was less than 4 months of age and involved the face, feet, ears, ventrum, axillary and inguinal regions, and perineum. The pruritus was nonseasonal, but was worse indoors, in the evenings, and in the morning. The dog sleeps in bed with the owners. The pruritus was only mildly responsive to oral antibiotics but was responsive to glucocorticoids; however, pruritus always returned when the glucocorticoids were discontinued. The owners practice flea control, and they have no other pets. The dog was acquired as a 4-month-old puppy from a pet store. At the time of presentation, the dog was receiving glucocorticoids (0.5 mg/kg PO q24h).

i. What is the major dermatological problem in this patient?

ii. List the differential diagnoses for this patient's dermatological problem. Some of these differential diagnoses are more likely than others; list them in order of importance giving explanations.

iii. What diagnostic tests should be recommended to the owner?

171 i. Pruritus.

ii. Lice and fleas are unlikely causes of the pruritus in this patient since the owners practice flea control, and the pattern and severity of the pruritus does not match that seen with flea or louse infestations. The pruritus associated with *Cheyletiella* is mild and dorsal in distribution, while this patient's pruritus is severe, and the pattern is ventral in distribution. Therefore, of the parasitic diseases in the differential diagnosis, *Sarcoptes* and *Demodex* are possible causes. *Demodex* should always be considered in the differential diagnosis of any dog with skin disease. Scabies is suspected in this patient because the dog was acquired from a pet store, the pruritus began at a young age, the pattern of the lesions and pruritus is ventral, the severity of the pruritus is severe, and the pruritus is worse at night. The latter three symptoms are very common in scabies patients.

Bacterial pyoderma, *Malassezia* dermatitis, and dermatophytosis should all be considered as possible causes for pruritus in this patient. A concurrent bacterial and yeast infection is highly probable, but this is most likely to be secondary to another disease. The fact that the lesions do not respond to antibiotics alone is consistent with a concurrent bacterial and yeast infection and/or an undiagnosed underlying trigger. Dermatophytosis should be included in the differential diagnosis because of the young age of onset, and the fact that the puppy was obtained from a pet store. What argues against dermatophytosis as a cause is that glucocorticoid administration did not worsen the lesions, and the owners have no history of having contracted a skin disease from their dog.

The pattern of lesions (face, feet, ears, ventrum) suggests that these infections were triggered by allergic skin disease. The two most likely allergic skin diseases are food allergy and atopy. The clinical signs are inconsistent with FAD; the pattern of FAD in dogs is caudal. Food allergy is more likely than atopy because of the young age of onset of the lesions. Atopy is still a reasonable differential diagnosis, especially a house dust mite allergy, because of the young age of onset, and the fact that the lesions are worse indoors.

iii. The diagnostic tests include: skin scrapings, a treatment trial for scabies, impression smears for yeast and bacteria and/or a 30 day treatment trial with anti-microbials, and a dermatophyte culture. A food trial and an intradermal skin test or *in vitro* allergy test may be necessary if the above diagnostics are negative or normal.

172 The patient in 171 presented with almost classic signs of atopy, yet intradermal skin testing (IDST) was delayed.
i. Why was IDST delayed in this patient?
ii. Would an *in vitro* diagnostic test for food allergy and/or atopy have been helpful at the first visit?
iii. What variations must a veterinarian be aware of with respect to commercially available *in vitro* allergy tests?

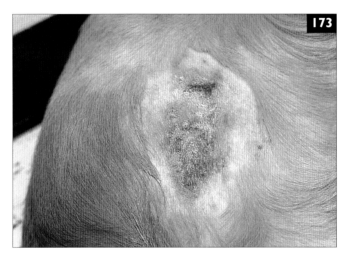

173 The lesion on the lumbosacral area of a dog shown (173) was initially diagnosed as an area of pyotraumatic dermatitis secondary to a flea infestation. The lesion was treated with a course of oral antibiotics and topical antibiotic ointment for 30 days. The lesion did not respond to therapy. What skin tumor of dogs can appear to be similar to an area of pyotraumatic dermatitis?

172 i. Intradermal skin testing was delayed in this patient for several reasons. First, the dog was receiving glucocorticoids at the time and an adequate withdrawal period (>6 weeks) was needed before testing. Second, the dog had severe secondary skin infections that needed to be resolved. Although atopy was considered a likely cause of the pruritus, it was unclear if this dog truly had year round pruritus. Dogs with seasonal atopy that develop secondary bacterial and/or yeast infections that are left untreated, can mimic year round pruritic dogs. It is always important to know whether or not the patient is still pruritic once the infections resolve. In addition, IDST is best delayed in patients with inflamed skin to avoid false positive reactions. Third, the onset of symptoms started at 4 months of age; most atopic dogs develop symptoms between 18 months to 7 years of age. *Sarcoptes scabiei* and a food allergy were the more likely differential diagnoses considering the age of onset in this patient. Fourth, the time of the year can impact on the results of IDST, especially in geographic regions with seasonal allergens. A negative result on the first IDST possibly occurred because the primary allergic disease was a food allergy and/or the dog had not been exposed to enough of the allergens to show positive reactions on the IDST. In this case, both of these were true.

ii. Because *in vitro* blood allergy tests are not reliable, restricted diet trials of 4–12 weeks are currently the only reliable method for diagnosing a food allergy. An *in vitro* blood allergy test for environmental allergens could have been done at the first visit; however, the question would still remain as to how the results should be interpreted. *In vitro* blood allergy tests and intradermal skin tests do not answer the question as to whether the patient is atopic or not. Instead, they establish which environmental allergens the patient reacts to. These tests (IDST or *in vitro* allergy tests) identify environmental allergens that will be used in formulating immunotherapy.

iii. Variations among tests may include source of allergen extract, reacting phase of the allergen (solid phase or liquid phase), specificity of the IgE detection reagent (some reagents may be contaminated with cross-reacting antibodies, i.e. IgG), signal molecule (enzyme-linked immunosorbant assay or radioallergosorbent test), sample processing (some laboratories pre-treat samples to remove nonIgE antibodies), reporting and interpretation of results (test results are not quantitatively reported), and standardization and quality control measures are voluntary in many countries (DeBoer and Hilliar, 2001).

173 Apocrine gland carcinoma may look similar to pyotraumatic dermatitis. In this case, the lack of response to what appeared to be appropriate therapy should alert the clinician that the dog has a different skin disease. The lack of response to appropriate therapy is one of the most important criteria for performing a skin biopsy.

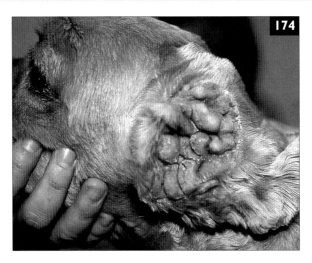

174 A 2-year-old cocker spaniel dog was presented for recurrent otitis externa. The opening to the external ear canal could not be found, and the vertical ear canal was hard upon palpation (174). Dermatological examination was normal except for nasal digital hyperkeratosis and mild scaling on the skin.
i. What common clinical syndrome is being depicted?
ii. What is the most likely underlying cause in this patient?
iii. How is this condition treated?

175 A 10-year-old male Labrador retriever dog was presented for evaluation of vomiting, diarrhea, and weight loss. In addition, the dog had numerous nonhealing draining lesions on the legs. A diagnosis of zygomycosis was made via intestinal biopsy.
i. What is zygomycosis and what are the most common clinical presentations of this disease?
ii. What organisms cause this disease?
iii. How is this disease diagnosed and what is unique about specimen handling?

174 i. Proliferative otitis externa.

ii. The most likely cause in a 2-year-old cocker spaniel dog is a primary disorder of keratinization. The nasal digital hyperkeratosis and scaling in the hair coat are also compatible with a disorder of keratinization.

iii. There are several treatment options, and the goal of therapy is to reestablish an open vertical and horizontal ear canal. Palpation of the ear canal may be all that is required to determine that the canal is calcified. In other cases, a skull radiograph should be taken to determine if there is calcification in the soft tissue of the ear canal, and/or to determine if the proliferative otitis is limited to the pinnae. If no calcification is present, systemic glucocorticoid therapy (2.2 mg/kg PO q24h for 3–4 weeks) may shrink this tissue and reestablish an open ear canal. If the ear tissue responds to systemic glucocorticoids, topical daily glucocorticoid otic preparations can be used to maintain the patency of the ear canal, especially in dogs with mild proliferative otitis. Alternatively, oral cyclosporin A (5 mg/kg q12h) for 12 weeks may be another option. If the proliferative tissue is limited to the pinnae, laser therapy can be used to remove the polyp-like tissue. If there is no response to glucocorticoid therapy or if calcification of the ear canal is present, the ears are considered 'end stage' and total ear canal ablation is the best surgical option. It is important for owners to understand that dogs with proliferative otitis externa due to a disorder of keratinization will be predisposed to further episodes and may eventually require surgery. Although the owners are focused on the ears, it is important that they understand the dog's generalized seborrhea will need to be treated and will require life-long therapy. Frequent bathing (2–3 times a week) is needed in many cases to treat dogs with severe primary disorders of keratinization.

175 i. Zygomycosis is a fungal disease caused by saprophytes that live in the soil or decaying vegetation. Affected animals may present with gastrointestinal, respiratory, or cutaneous lesions. Single or multiple wounds, or nonhealing wounds characterize the cutaneous presentations.

ii. Zygomyocetes are are divided into two orders: Muorales (*Rhizopus*, *Mucor*, or *Absida*, and *Mortierella*) and Enomophthorales (*Conidiobolus* and *Basidobolus*).

iii. Definitive diagnosis is made via biopsy and culture. Characteristic biopsy findings include diffuse, pyogranulomatus to granulomatous inflammation. Eosinophils are often prominent. The inflammation tends to be centered around amorphous eosinophilic material and poorly staining fungal hyphae are often seen. Fungal elements are usually found within foci of necrosis. The organism can be cultured on Sabouraud's dextrose agar by embedding a wedge of tissue into the media without cycloheximide. It is important not to macerate the tissue as this may destroy the organism.

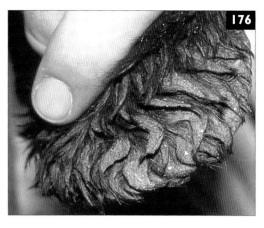

176 The ear margin of a 3-year-old springer spaniel dog is shown (176). The owners report that this material accumulates on the ear margin within 2–3 days after bathing. The ear margins are matted with greasy accumulations of follicular casts adhering to the skin and to the hair. The remainder of the dog's skin is normal. Skin scrapings are negative, and previous impression smears of the exudate revealed poorly staining ceruminous debris, with some cocci and *Malassezia* organisms. The dog has been treated with oral antibiotics and concurrent ketoconazole several times previously, but the condition always recurs.

i. What is the clinical diagnosis, and how should the dog be treated?
ii. Ear margin dermatoses are common in which dog breed(s), and how do lesions progress?

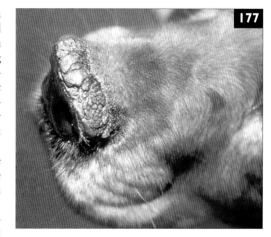

177 The dorsal planum of a 2-year-old female cocker spaniel dog is shown (177). This lesion started to develop when the dog was <1 year of age. Physical examination reveals hyperkeratotic footpads, follicular fronds surrounding her mammae, and mildly malodorous ears with a thick yellow discharge.

i. What is the clinical name for the condition described? What is the etiology? How is this condition managed?
ii. If these lesions occurred suddenly in an older dog, what could be the cause?
iii. What skin disease has been described recently in Labrador retriever dogs that appears similar to this one?

176, 177: Answers

176 i. Ear margin seborrhea/dermatosis complicated by secondary bacterial and yeast pyoderma. Ear margin seborrhea can be the only clinical manifestation of primary seborrhea in some dogs. If this is the case, the condition is best managed by close clipping of the hair coat, and frequent bathing of the ear margins several times a week with an antiseborrheic shampoo. Close clipping of the hair coat facilitates the bathing.
ii. Ear margin dermatosis is common in dachshunds and other breeds with pendulous ears. The clinical signs consist of follicular casts matting the hair and plugging hair follicles. As the disorder progresses, the scaling starts to involve the entire ear margin, resulting in any combination of inflammation, hair loss and/or thickening of margin. Advanced lesions can lead to head shaking and the development of fissures and crusts. The ear margin is notorious for poor healing, and some patients require extensive surgical debridement (i.e. ear cropping) to arrest fissuring. Laser surgery can be very helpful in these cases.

177 i. Nasal digital hyperkeratosis. The young age of the dog and the other clinical findings suggest that this dog has a primary disorder of keratinization. Such dogs develop a wide spectrum of clinical diseases, and dogs with nasal hyperkeratosis can be managed but not cured. If the lesions are mild, they should be hydrated for 5–10 minutes and treated with a keratolytic agent such as tretinoin gel. This will need to be done daily until the nose (and footpads) is normal and repeated as needed. If there is severe fissuring and/or hyperkeratosis, the excess keratin should be surgically trimmed first. This is best done under sedation by a clinician. The author finds it helpful to hydrate the tissues for 10–15 minutes prior to trimming the keratin. Care must be taken not to be too aggressive since a normal amount of keratin is needed to protect the nose and footpads. In some patients, white petroleum jelly can be applied to hydrated tissue to soften the lesions.
ii. The acute onset of nasal and/or footpad crusting should make the clinician suspicious of PF, lupus erythematosus, and hepatocutaneous syndrome. Other differential diagnoses for nasal hyperkeratosis include zinc responsive dermatosis and ichthyosis, usually diseases of younger, healthy dogs.
iii. Hereditary nasal parakeratosis in Labrador retriever dogs (Page *et al.*, 2003). This is an inherited disorder with an autosomal recessive mode of inheritance. Lesions are often first seen between 6 and 12 months of age and start as mounds of hyperkeratosis on the dorsal aspect of the nasal planum. The severity varies, with some dogs having only small amounts of brownish dry keratin on their nose while others develop severe fissures and erosions. Histologically, this syndrome is characterized by parakeratotic hyperkeratosis. Dogs with this condition do not respond well to systemic therapies and the lesions are managed medically with topical emollients such as vitamin E, petroleum jelly, and propylene glycol.

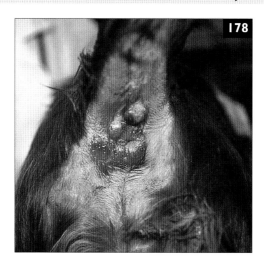

178 A dog was presented as an after-hours emergency for the complaint of acute rectal bleeding. Note the perianal furunculosis, erythema, and exudation (**178**). After sedation, fistulous tracts were found 1–2 cm lateral to the anus in positions between 6 and 8 o'clock.
i. What is the diagnosis?
ii. How should the dog be treated?
iii. What is the source of secretions of the anal sac and what is its function?

179 A Wood's lamp is an ultra-violet light with a wavelength of 253.7 nm that is filtered through a cobalt or nickel filter. It is used as a screening tool in the diagnosis of dermatophytosis (**179**).

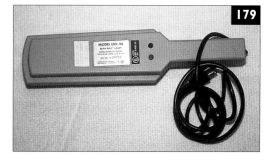

i. What is the principle of its use, and how is the lamp prepared for use?
ii. What are the common mistakes made in interpretation of results?
iii. What species of dermatophytes does it screen for?

178 i. Anal sac abscessation with rupture and perineal furunculosis.
ii. This is a chronic problem due to extensive perianal furunculosis and cellulitis. Under general anesthesia, all of the hair from the surrounding area should be clipped. The abscesses should be incised and debrided by curettage, and the wounds should be flushed with a large volume of a dilute antibacterial solution (povidone-iodine or chlorhexidine). Appropriate analgesic treatment should be prescribed, as home care will require twice-daily hydrotherapy. Oral antibiotics (e.g. cephalexin 30 mg/kg PO q12h for 30 days) should be prescribed. Healing of the lesions will occur by granulation. There is the risk that damage to the anal sacs and/or ducts may lead to chronic fistulous tracts and recurrent infections. If this occurs, surgical removal of the anal sacs may be necessary. In this dog, the diffuse perianal furunculosis suggests that there may be an underlying pruritic trigger. Surgical excision may resolve the infections, but relapses of perianal furunculosis and inflammation will persist unless the underlying cause is found.
iii. The walls of the sac are comprised of sebaceous glands and the ducts are lined with numerous epitrichial sweat glands. The anal sac fluid is a mixture of fatty acids, serous secretions, and cellular debris. The function is unknown but is presumed to be part of scent marking/social function.

179 i. The Wood's lamp is a screening tool for dermatophytes that produce a fluorescing metabolite as they grow on hairs. This metabolite is only produced on growing hairs. The Wood's lamp should be turned on for at least 5 minutes prior to use. The stability of the wavelength and its intensity are temperature dependent. The animal should be placed in a dark room and the light held over suspect lesions for 3–5 minutes. Some dermatophytes are slow to show the apple-green fluorescence. In addition, it takes several minutes for the clinician's eyes to adapt to the dark, allowing them to see the fluorescence.
ii.. The Wood's lamp is suggestive, but not diagnostic of a dermatophyte infection. Glowing hairs should be cultured to confirm the infection. These hairs can also be examined with a clearing agent to look for the presence of fungal spores and hyphae on or in hairs. Topical medications and shampoos can cause false positives or destroy the fluorescence altogether. Keratin, sebum, and bacterial organisms will also glow. True fluorescence is present only on hairs. If the distal portion of the hair glows, the hair should be plucked to see if the proximal portion (intrafollicular) also glows.
iii. Only a limited number of dermatophytes produce fluorescence: *Microsporum canis*, *M. distortum*, *M. audouinii*, and *Trichophyton schoeleinni*. The only pathogen of veterinary importance that glows is *M. canis* and not all strains fluoresce. It has been estimated that only 50% of strains of *M. canis* fluoresce.

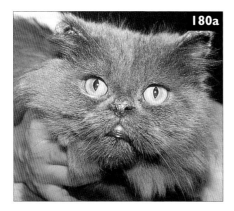

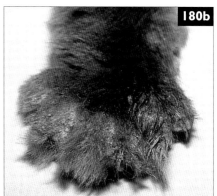

180 An adult Persian-mix cat was presented for examination of resistant *Microsporum canis* infection. The breeder, who had had several cats before with dermatophytosis, made this diagnosis. The cat started to develop skin lesions several months ago, and she treated the cat topically with twice weekly lime sulfur rinses. After several months of treatment, the cat was still developing lesions and was presented for examination. Dermatological examination revealed thick adherent crusting on the nose, ear tips, and footpads

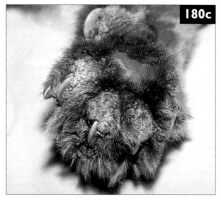

(180a–c). Small crusts could be palpated in the hair coat, and careful examination of the cat revealed intact pustules around the nipples. The owner reported the cat was intermittently depressed, and today the cat was depressed and had a fever.
i. What are the two most likely differential diagnoses? Which is the most likely diagnosis?
ii. What diagnostic tests should be performed?
iii. How is this disease treated, and what is the prognosis?

181 A dog is presented with firm, hard, painful footpads. There are areas of ulceration with a discharge consisting of a white chalky material. Histological findings reveal calcinosis cutis.
i. What is the most likely cause of the cutaneous calcinosis cutis?
ii. What is calcinosis circumscripta?

180 i. Facial and footpad crusting (pododermatitis) in cats is most commonly caused by dermatophytosis or PF. However, the most likely diagnosis in this cat is PF. There is no hair loss as expected in dermatophytosis, and the intact pustules found near the nipples are a classic finding in feline PF.

ii. Skin scrapings of the exudates from the footpads should be obtained to rule out mites. Even though dermatophytosis is unlikely, a fungal culture should be performed to eliminate this cause, and to make sure it is not now a concurrent skin disease. Early cases of PF in cats can look surprisingly similar to dermatophytosis. Even though it is difficult to biopsy the fragile pustules found in feline PF, an elliptical skin biopsy using a scalpel blade should be used to harvest an intact pustule from the nipple area. Skin biopsy punch instruments are best avoided because they may rupture the fragile pustules. The pustule should be carefully collected and mounted subcutaneous side down on a piece of a wooden tongue depressor. If there are multiple intact pustules, several should be submitted for examination. Lastly, impression smears of the exudates from the foot pads, underside of the crusts on the ear, and pustules should be made to look for cytological evidence of PF, i.e. acantholytic cells.

iii. This is a case of PF in a cat. It is an autoimmune skin disease that requires life-long therapy, although some cats may have remissions of several months' duration. Cats are often treated with a combination of glucocorticoids, chlorambucil, and gold salts. The author has managed many cats with injectable triamcinolone acetate as sole therapy. Azathioprine is toxic in cats and should not be used. The prognosis for a good quality of life is high.

181 i. The most likely cause is metastatic calcinosis cutis. Calcinosis cutis is most commonly associated with hyperadrenocorticism; calcium deposits can occur anywhere but are most common on the dorsum and in the axillae and groin. Calcium deposits solely in the footpads are rare and are most commonly associated with dogs with chronic renal disease or in young dogs with renal dysplasia. Calcinosis cutis is a clinical manifestation of a systemic disease. The underlying cause of calcinosis cutis is determined by history, physical examination findings, and laboratory tests

ii. Calcinosis circumscripta is a localized form of dystrophic calcification in areas of previous trauma (pressure points, bite wounds, ear croppings). The cause is unknown. Lesions occur in young dogs and are dome shaped, firm or fluctuant, ulcerated or haired.

182 A 4-year-old male cat was presented for 'feline hyperesthesia syndrome'. The cat was growling, overgrooming, and biting itself. The neurology service requested a derma-tological examination because the cat's symp-toms did not respond to phenobarbital or diaze-

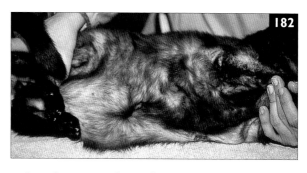

pam, but the lesions did respond to glucocorticoids. Further questioning of the owner revealed the cat had been symptomatic for 3 years. The symptoms occurred year round but were clearly worse in the fall and again at Christmas time. The owners always had a fresh cut Christmas tree, and the cat spent a lot of time in and around the tree. The most dramatic dermatological finding was patchy hair loss characterized by short broken hairs that appeared to be chewed off and 'twitching and biting of the skin' when scratched (182). Other dermatological findings included scattered erythematous papules, linear excoriations in the pre-auricular area, patchy hyperpigmentation in the inner pinnae, broken and bent whiskers, black debris at the nail base, scales pierced by hairs throughout the coat, and broken and frayed nails. Two other cats in the house were normal. The people had no skin lesions.

i. What is this cat's primary dermatological problem?
ii. What are the most likely differential diagnoses?
iii. Based upon the information presented, what are the possible working diagnoses?
iv. What is the most likely reason the cat becomes more symptomatic at Christmas time?

183 The focal area of hair loss shown is darkly pigmented (183). Upon closer examination, diffuse follicular plugging is causing the skin pigmen-tation. This 'gray' discolored lesion is very typical of a common skin disease seen in dogs, especially puppies. What is it?

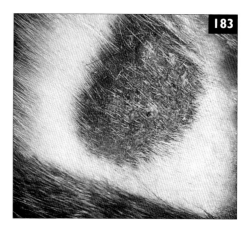

182 i. Generalized pruritus. The cat's clinical signs and history are not compatible with feline hyperesthesia syndrome. In feline hyperesthesia, affected cats violently groom and self-mutilate themselves in random, unpredictable, explosive attacks. They often growl, vocalize, run, and may attack others. Owners describe the cats acting as if they are in pain. The skin over the dorsum of the back may twitch or ripple just prior to an episode.
ii. The most common causes of generalized pruritus in cats include: parasitic diseases (fleas, lice, *Cheyletiella* and *Demodex* mites), infections (bacterial and/or yeast pyoderma, dermatophytosis), and allergic skin diseases (atopy, food allergy, flea allergy). Several key historical points help limit the differential diagnoses. First, two other cats in the house are normal making a contagious or infectious skin disease unlikely (i.e. fleas, lice, *Cheyletiella*, contagious feline demodicosis, and dermatophytosis). Second, the response to glucocorticoids suggests an underlying cause is more likely to be an allergic disease rather than a contagious or infectious disease. Third, the owners have no lesions making contagious mites and fleas unlikely. Finally, although the symptoms are year round, there are two points in the year where seasonal spikes are observed (fall and Christmas time).
iii. There are four possible working diagnoses. First, this cat could have year round pruritus due to a food allergy and seasonal atopy. Second, it could have year round pruritus due to a food allergy and year round atopy that happens to have seasonal spikes. Third, it could just have year round atopy with seasonal spikes. Finally, the cat could have seasonal atopy and untreated/unrecognized complicating secondary bacterial and/or yeast infections giving the impression that the pruritus is year round.
This cat was examined in January after the owner had removed the Christmas tree. Large numbers of *Malassezia* spp. were found in cytological examinations of the black nail bed debris scraped from beneath the cat's nails. The scaling with hairs piercing the scales was compatible with a bacterial infection. The cat's pruritus resolved with 35 days of oral antibiotic and antifungal therapy. The cat remained normal until the fall when it exhibited signs of pruritus. The episode was managed with alternate day glucocorticoid therapy. The owners bought an artificial Christmas tree, and the cat did not relapse during the holiday season.
iv. Atopic dogs and cats often become more pruritic during Christmas time if owners have a fresh cut tree in their home. Relapses are triggered by the sudden concentration of pollen.

183 This common skin disease is demodicosis. *Demodex* mites live in the hair follicles; when they proliferate they plug the follicles, impeding the release of sebum from the sebaceous glands. Clinically this appears as a focal area of gray pigmentation. The surface of the skin is often waxy.

184 A 2-year-old spayed female samoyed dog was presented for the problem of hair loss that spared the dog's head and legs. Physical examination revealed noninflammatory hairloss on the dog's trunk, ventral chest, and caudal thighs (184). The dog was polyuric and polydipsic, but not pruritic. All other diagnostics were normal or negative. Skin biopsies were compatible with an endocrine alopecia. The results of the thyroid and adrenal function testing are shown.

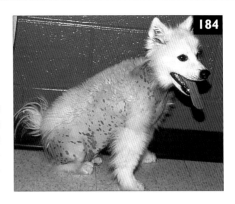

	Results	Normal
Total thyroxine (TT4) nmol/l	30	15–67
Total triiodothyronine (TT3) nmol/l	1.4	1.0–2.5
Free T4 by dialysis pmol/l	8	6–42
Free (unbound) T3 (FT3) pmol/l	6.5	4.0–12.0
T4 autoantibody	5	<20
T3 autoantibody	0	<10
Thyroid stimulating hormone mU/L	15	0–37
Thyroglobuline autoantibody %	11	<200

Low-dose dexamethasone suppression test (ng/ml)	Results	Normal
Pre-	84	2.1–58.8
4 hr	7	<10
8 hr	6	<10

ACTH stimulation test (ng/ml)	Results	Normal
Pre-	45	2.1–58
Post-	80	65.0–174

Adrenal function panel clinical endocrinology service/University of Tennessee, Tennessee USA

	Result (baseline)	Normal range	Result (post-ACTH)	Normal range
Cortisol ng/ml	152.4	2.1–58.8	159.7	65.0–174.6
Androstenedione ng/ml	21.2	0.1–5.7	29.5	2.7–39.7
Estrogen	60.4	30.8–69.9	51.5	27.9–69.2
Progesterone ng/ml	1.83	0.01–0.49	2.15	0.10–1.50
17-OH Progesterone ng/ml	1.98	0.01–0.77	2.63	0.40–1.62
Testosterone ng/ml	<0.01	0.01–0.32	0.01	0.02–0.45

i. What is the interpretation of the ACTH stimulation, low-dose dexamethasone suppression, and thyroid function tests?

ii. An adrenal panel test was performed several months later. What is the most likely diagnosis? What are the characteristics of the disease that the adrenal panel is screening for?

184 i. When interpreted as a whole, the thyroid hormone screening panel indicated normal function. The ACTH stimulation test indicated an elevated basal cortisol concentration, but when stimulated the dog was within the normal range. The low-dose dexamethasone suppression test revealed an elevated basal cortisol, but suppression was normal. At this point, hypothyroidism and hyperadrenocorticism were unlikely, but there did appear to be increased adrenal activity.

ii. The findings were compatible with increased adrenal activity. At this time, the dog had a markedly increased basal cortisol, but again the dog's post-ACTH stimulation test was within laboratory normals. There was also an increased basal androstenedione and increased pre- and post-ACTH progesterone and 17-OH progesterone. These findings were most compatible with adrenal hyperplasia-like syndrome; however, an adrenal tumor should not be ruled out based upon these findings. An abdominal ultrasound was normal, and the final diagnosis was adrenal hyperplasia-like disorder (alopecia X).

This is an endocrine disorder of dogs characterized by coat changes and hair loss that starts between 1 and 2 years of age. The earliest clinical signs are a gradual dulling of the hair coat, dry hair coat, and loss of primary hairs. Hair loss starts in the frictional areas of the tail head, caudal thigh region, and caudomedial thigh and collar region. The head and extremities are spared. Polyuria and polydipsia can be seen as in hyperadrenocorticism and diabetes mellitus, but are usually not as severe. Studies on dogs with this syndrome showed they have either elevated baseline and/or post-ACTH concentrations of sex hormones, especially progesterones. The most commonly affected breeds are pomeranians, chow chows, keeshonds, and samoyeds. The diagnosis is made by history, clinical signs, ruling out other causes of hair loss, particularly endocrine diseases and follicular dysplasia, and by specialized pre- and post-ACTH sex hormone assays. A skin biopsy should be performed to rule out hair follicle dysplasia and to confirm the hair loss is due to an endocrine disorder. Hypothyroidism should be ruled out as an underlying cause. Both an ACTH stimulation test and a low-dose dexamethasone suppression test are recommended to rule out hyperadrenocorticism. If these are normal then an adrenal sex hormone panel is indicated. In some dogs with chronic disease, there may be elevations in pre- and post-ACTH stimulation cortisol concentrations. Therefore, a low-dose dexamethasone suppression test should be done as part of the diagnostic evaluation. Currently, the only reliable diagnostic laboratory performing adrenal sex hormone testing is the Endocrinology Laboratory at the University of Tennessee, College of Veterinary Medicine, Knoxville TN.

185 The chin of an 11-year-old male black Labrador retriever dog is shown (185).
i. What condition is being depicted?
ii. What is poliosis?

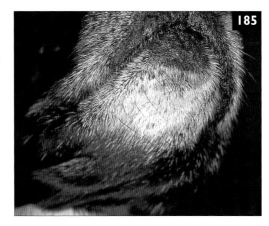

186 A 3-year-old female Siberian husky dog is presented for the complaint of 'crusties'. The owner reports the dog has pruritic crusty lesions on the face and ears. On dermatological examination, the lesions around the eyes are symmetrical (186), and similar lesions are present on the ear margins, chin, ears, footpads, and pressure points. The skin is thickened and hyperkeratotic crusting is present. The dog is healthy otherwise. The dog is fed a complete and balanced diet. Two littermates, owned by other people, have similar lesions.

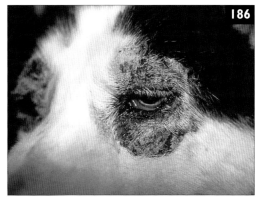

i. What is the most likely diagnosis and how should this be confirmed?
ii. How should the dog be treated, and how soon would resolution of clinical signs be expected?
iii. What endocrine disease may play a role in the pathogenesis of this disease?

187 What are oomycete infections?

185 i. The condition shown is graying of the hair coat due to age. Depigmentation of the hair coat is called leukotrichia.
ii. Poliosis is premature graying of hair.

186 i. Zinc-responsive skin disease. The signalment, clinical signs, and affected littermates are compatible with zinc deficiency The diagnosis could be confirmed by skin biopsy. The key finding is diffuse parakeratosis, especially of the follicular epithelium. Serum and hair concentrations of zinc may be abnormal, but it is difficult to find a reliable laboratory to do the testing. Siberian husky, Alaskan malamute and some bull terrier dogs have an inherited defect that decreases their capability to absorb zinc from the intestines. This is called syndrome I of zinc-responsive skin diseases. Syndrome II occurs in rapidly growing dogs that are fed zinc deficient diets high in phytates or minerals (e.g. calcium), or diets oversupplemented with minerals and vitamins that interfere with zinc absorption.
ii. This dog needs 1 mg/kg of elemental zinc each day. The most commonly used supplements are zinc sulfate (10 mg/kg/day), zinc gluconate (5 mg/kg/day), or zinc methionine (1.7 mg/kg/day). Feeding a dog food with 'zinc' is not adequate nor are vitamin supplements containing zinc. Some Siberian husky dogs do not respond to oral supplementation and may require intravenous injections of zinc sulfate solutions (10–15 mg/kg) weekly for at least 4 weeks, and then every 1–6 months thereafter. Therapy is life-long. Improvement in clinical signs is usually evident within a few weeks. After the diagnosis, the lesions should be hydrated and the crusts soaked off.
iii. Thyroid hormones are important in the absorption and utilization of zinc. Dogs that develop spontaneously occurring hypothyroidism may develop clinical and histological signs of zinc-responsive skin disease. These dogs may fail to respond to zinc supplementation if their hypothyroidism is not diagnosed and treated.

187 Oomycete infections are caused by aquatic pathogens of the protoctistid class oomycetes. These organisms are found in wet tropical and subtropical climates and infection is caused by exposure and/or consumption of contaminated water. The organisms exist as motile zoospores that show chemotaxis toward damaged plants or animal tissues. Phythiosis is caused by *Phythium insidiosum* and has three clinical presentations: gastrointestinal, subcutaneous, and nasopharyngeal. Recently a new organism, *Lagenidium*, has been identified in this class and is associated with cutaneous and/or subcutaneous lesions as well as systemic lesions. Treatment for both diseases is difficult and prognosis is grave.

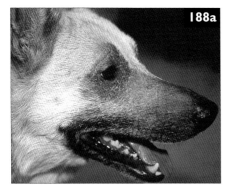
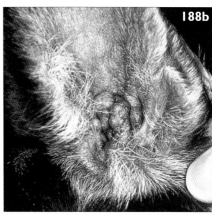

188 A 3-year-old male castrated police dog was presented for a second opinion (188a). The dog had been diagnosed with year round atopic dermatitis and had face, muzzle, periocular, and otic erythema, and hair loss at the time of examination. The police officer who owned the dog was very willing to carry out immunotherapy for the treatment of the dog's atopic dermatitis. The reason, however, for the second opinion was the dog had bilateral proliferative otitis externa, and the dog's hearing was impaired. The previous veterinarian had radiographed the dog's skull and determined the vertical and horizontal ear canals were completely obstructed by soft tissue (188b). Bilateral ear canal ablations were recommended to resolve this situation. The dog's function was impaired in its current state and surgical treatment would not return the dog to normal function. The owner is inquiring if there is any other treatment option. On examination of the radiographs, no evidence of soft tissue calcification is seen. What other treatment options are available, if any?

189 A kitten was born dead to a queen treated with griseofulvin for dermatophytosis during the first trimester of her pregnancy (189).
i. What is the most likely cause of the kitten's death?
ii. What is the mechanism of action of griseofulvin?
iii. How is the drug absorbed and delivered to the skin?

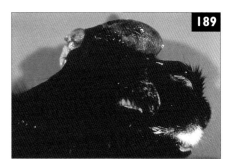

188 Proliferative ear tissue is often very responsive to glucocorticoid therapy. The proliferative tissue often shrinks when the patient is treated with oral glucocorticoids. If adequate patency of the ear canal is obtained, the proliferative tissue can often be controlled with ear cleaning and continued administration of topical otic glucocorticoids. The lack of calcification of the ear tissue makes this dog a good candidate for this therapy. The patient was treated with prednisone (1 mg/kg PO q24h) for 15 days and then every other day for an additional 15 days. The proliferative tissue regressed, and the

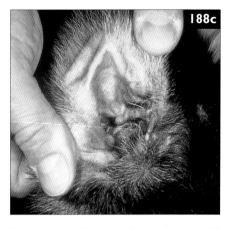

ear canal regained normal patency (188c). Concurrent topical steroids and successful immunotherapy were able to maintain normal patency of the dog's ear canals. For dogs that cannot tolerate prednisone therapy, cyclosporin A therapy is another option (5 mg/kg PO q12h for up to 12 weeks).

189 i. This kitten died as a result of a griseofulvin-induced birth defect. Griseofulvin is a known teratogen and should not be administered to pregnant cats. Pregnant queens cannot be safely treated with any of the commonly used systemic antifungal agents. Topical therapy with lime sulfur (sponge-on dips twice weekly) is recommended as a safe alternative therapy.
ii. Griseofulvin is a fungistatic antifungal drug produced by *Penicillium griseofulvum*. It works by inhibition of cell wall synthesis, nucleic acid synthesis, and mitotis. It is primarily active against growing organisms, but it may keep dormant cells from dividing. Griseofulvin inhibits nucleic acid synthesis and cell mitosis by arresting division at metaphase, interfering with the function of spindle microtubules, morphogenetic changes in fungal cells, and possibly interfering with chitin synthesis.
iii. Griseofulvin is not well absorbed from the gastrointestinal tract, and should be administered with a fatty meal to enhance absorption. Since particle size also affects absorption of the drug, it is formulated in a microsize and ultramicrosize formulation. The drug can be detected in the stratum corneum within 8 hours to 3 days of administration. The highest concentrations are in the stratum corneum. The drug is delivered to the stratum corneum by diffusion, sweating, and transepidermal fluid loss. It is deposited in keratin precursor cells and remains there throughout the differentiation process. Griseofulvin concentrations drop rapidly after discontinuation of therapy, as it is not tightly bound to keratin.

190 A 4-year-old great Dane dog was presented for a second opinion for resistant dermatophytosis. According to the medical record, a dermatophyte culture was performed on one of the multifocal areas of hair loss (**190**). The fungal culture was recorded as 'positive' because the DTM turned red. However, there was no microscopic confirmation of dermatophytosis. The dog was treated with griseofulvin (50 mg/kg PO

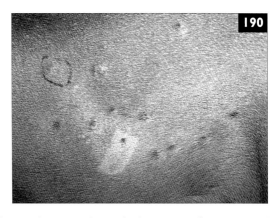

q24h) for the last 6 weeks. The lesions have not diminished in size or frequency and may be spreading. On examination today, multifocal areas of hair loss can be found. The hairs are not broken or frayed but shed completely. The lesions are Wood's lamp negative, and skin scrapings are negative for *Demodex* mites. This dog has a common skin disease that is often confused with dermatophytosis. What disease does it have?

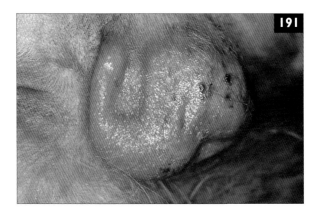

191 An intact male golden retriever dog is presented for examination before placement in foster care prior to adoption. It is thin, but otherwise appears healthy. During the examination, matted hair from around the prepuce and scrotal area was clipped and a scrotal ulceration found (**191**). The dog has a nice temperament but is not easily controlled.
i. What are the differential diagnoses for scrotal ulceration in dogs?
ii. How should the veterinarian proceed?

190 i. Bacterial pyoderma; these lesions are frequently misdiagnosed as 'ringworm' lesions. The dermatophyte culture in this dog was incompletely evaluated. The red color indicator on DTM is not diagnostic of dermatophyte growth, it only indicates that the organism seen is using the protein in the medium. Definitive diagnosis of a dermatophyte culture requires microscopic identification of the colony growth (i.e. confirmation of the identity of the dermatophyte). The dog's lesions resolved completely with a 21 day course of oral antibiotics.

191 i. The causes of scrotal ulceration in the dog are numerous and include, but are not limited to: BP, drug eruptions, erythema multiforme, lupus erythematosus, pemphigus vulgaris or PF, irritant or allergic skin disease, bacterial pyoderma, self-trauma, yeast dermatitis, canine babesiosis, leishmaniasis, and canine Rocky Mountain spotted fever (*Rickettsia rickettsia*).
ii. This patient requires a careful and thorough re-examination, particularly of mucocutaneous regions. In addition, it is necessary to biopsy suspect skin lesions rather rapidly as vesicles, bulla, and pustules are fragile and transient. Finally, scrotal ulceration is very painful, and any diagnostic testing would be difficult to perform. Thus, chemical restraint is indicated in this patient. A careful examination of the oral cavity and all mucocutaneous junctions, axilla, and inguinal areas should be performed. Because immune-mediated diseases are suspect, any bullae, vesicles, or pustules should be biopsied immediately. Impression smears of the scrotal ulceration should be performed looking for cytological evidence of infection and/or microbial overgrowth. Serum and blood samples should be collected for antinuclear antibody testing and rickettsial diseases, and a complete blood count performed.

After sedating this patient, large numbers of small, but flaccid, intact pustules were found in the haired area bordering the scrotal ulceration. Impression smears revealed large numbers of degenerate neutrophils, cocci, and rafts of acanthocytes. A skin biopsy of the pustules was obtained. There was a delay of 14 days before a final diagnosis was made, pending laboratory test results. During this time, no treatment was prescribed (at the request of the rescue agency). The foster family reported the dog was intermittently depressed and febrile every 5–7 days. In addition, the hair coat became crusted and lesions developed on the face, inner pinnae, and footpads. The final diagnosis was PF.

Lesions in this dog began on the scrotum even though facial lesions and footpad crusting are often the first lesions seen in this disease. This disease is treated most commonly with glucocorticoids and concurrent immunosuppressive drugs, e.g. gold salts and azathioprine.

192 The footpad of a 6-month-old stray puppy found in Texas, near the USA–Mexico border is shown (192). Careful examination revealed a small amount of nasal hyperkeratosis in addition to small amounts of ocular and nasal discharge, and a fever.

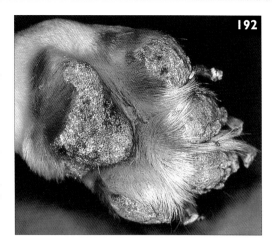

i. What are the differential diagnoses for nasal digital hyperkeratosis?
ii. Which of these differential diagnoses is the most likely cause of the digital hyperkeratosis?

193 A 5-year-old female cocker spaniel dog is presented for treatment of a chronic skin disease of 1 year's duration. The owner reports the dog gradually developed crusting, dark skin, and scales in her hair coat. She also described the skin as having 'scales that stick out of hair follicles making the dog look like she has fish scales'. The axillary area of the dog is shown (193). Note the hyperpigmentation caused by follicular plugging and hyperkeratotic plaques. Follicular fronds are also present throughout the coat, giving the dog the 'fish scale appearance' the owner mentioned. The erythema is suggestive of a bacterial infection.

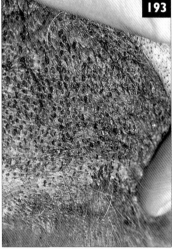

i. What is follicular plugging? Marked follicular plugging occurs most commonly in which skin diseases?
ii. Skin scrapings were negative, and the dog was otherwise healthy. This dog's lesions did not respond completely to a course of antibiotics and topical antiseborrheic therapy. What is the next diagnostic step?
iii. What are retinoids, what is their proposed mechanism of action, what diseases are they used to treat, and what adverse effects do they cause?

194 What is swimmer's itch?

192 i. The common causes of nasal digital hyperkeratosis include zinc deficiency, leishmaniasis, primary disorder of keratinization, drug eruptions, PF, lupus erythematosus, hepatocutaneous syndrome, and canine distemper virus.
ii. The vaccination history of this puppy is unknown, and the dog is showing signs of systemic illness; therefore, distemper is the most likely cause. Canine distemper is endemic in this region of the USA.

193 i. Follicular plugging is an accumulation of keratin in the follicular ostium. Follicular plugging may be seen in hyperadrenocorticism, sebaceous adenitis, Vitamin A deficiency, hypervitaminosis A, generalized demodicosis, and follicular dysplasia.
ii. Skin biopsy. Vitamin A-responsive skin diseases, follicular dysplasia, and sebaceous adenititis are all diagnosed via skin biopsy. This is a case of vitamin A-responsive skin disease. This disease is most common in cocker spaniel dogs, and it is unknown if it is heritable. Skin biopsy findings revealed marked follicular orthokeratotic hyperkeratosis, with microscopic fronds of keratin oozing out of the hair follicle ostium. The dog responded to 10,000 IU of oral vitamin A with a fatty meal. Improvement was seen within a few weeks, but complete resolution of lesions took >8 weeks. Concurrent topical therapy with antiseborrheic shampoos every 2–3 days was also prescribed. Discontinuation of the oral vitamin A resulted in a relapse.
iii. Retinoids may be synthetic or naturally occurring drugs that have vitamin A activity. The synthetic retinoids include retinol, retinoic acid, and retinal derivatives. Retinoids have a wide range of biological actions including regulation of proliferation, growth, and differentiation of epithelial tissues. Retinoids are used in dermatology to treat disorders of keratinization. Adverse effects include keratoconjunctivitis sicca, decreased tear production, vomiting, diarrhea, stiffness, pruritus, and mucocutaneous erythema in dogs. Laboratory abnormalities include hypertriglyceridemia, hyperchlolesterolemia, and increased alanine animinotransferase, aspartate aminotransferase, and serum alkaline phosphatase. These drugs are also teratogenic.

194 Swimmer's itch is the common name for *Schistosoma* dermatitis. *Schistosoma* cercariae are parasites of ducks, shore birds, voles, mice, and muskrats. When the miracidia hatches it must find a natural host within 12 hours or die. In lakes heavily infested with this organism, people and their pets may become infested. Dogs show symptoms within 1 day of exposure. The lesions are intensely pruritic and may resemble mosquito, chigger, or fleabites. The author has seen several suspect cases of this disorder where both the dog and owner developed symptoms after swimming in a lake reported to have infestation with this parasite.

195 A 4-year-old female spayed Labrador retriever dog was presented for multiple cutaneous masses of 8 months' duration. Physical examination revealed multiple raised, firm, cutaneous masses in the dermis and subcutaneous tissue (195). The lesions were nonpruritic and haired. According to the owner, the lesions tend to wax and wane. The dog is otherwise healthy.

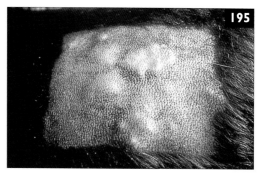

i. Nodules and tumors in dogs are classified as inflammatory (infectious and noninfectious) or neoplastic. What initial diagnostic tests are indicated in this case?
ii. List the noninfectious differential diagnoses for this dog's lesions.
iii. What advanced diagnostic testing techniques are available that enhance identification of various cell types from biopsy specimens?

196 A kitten is one of a litter of six presented for examination. The kittens were presented for scratching at their ears. Upon examination, there was black brown waxy debris in the ears (196a). A mite was found on the examination of an ear swab (196b).
i. What is the diagnosis?
ii. What is the recommended treatment?
iii. List three other pediatric diseases which can present with a similar appearance.

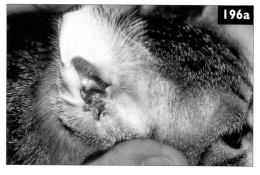

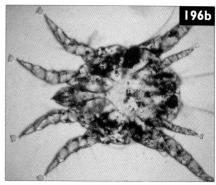

195 i. Initial diagnostic testing should include a skin biopsy, fine needle aspirate, cytological examination of cut sections of tissue, and tissue culture. Neoplasia is unlikely due to the age of the dog and overall good health. Thus, the most likely cause is an infectious disease. Cultures should be done on aseptically collected surgical specimens and submitted for aerobic, fungal, and mycobacteria cultures. After blotting the blood from a tissue specimen, multiple tissue imprints on a glass slide should be obtained and submitted, unfixed and unstained, to a diagnostic laboratory for acid-fast staining. Mycobacterial organisms are rare on histological sections but may be more numerous on cytological preparations.

This was a case of idiopathic sterile granuloma/pyogranuloma. The dog was treated with oral prednisone (2.2 mg/kg PO q24h) until the lesions resolved. Relapse is common in this disorder, and affected dogs may require intermittent life-long therapy. Refractory cases can be managed with azathioprine (2.2 mg/kg PO q24h).
ii. Noninfectious causes of nodules include urticaria, angioedema, eosinophilic granulomas, arthropod bite granulomas, calcinosis cutis, calcinosis circumscripta, xanthoma, panniculitis, hematomas, seroma, cutaneous amyloidosis, canine cellulitis, histiocytic diseases, nodular dermatofibrosis, sterile nodular granuloma and pyogranuloma, and foreign body reactions (Shearer and Dobson, 2002).
iii. Advanced diagnostic testing procedures routinely available for identification of various cell types in biopsy specimens include, but are not limited to: electron microscopy, immunostaining with polycolonal anti-*Mycobacterium bovis* (BCG), enzyme histochemistry, immunocytochemistry, and immunofluorescence testing. Anti-BCG testing immunohistostaining is useful for rapid identification of many infectious agents (bacterial, fungal, mycobacterial, and nocardial organisms).

196 i. *Otodectes cyanotis* (ear mites).
ii. The ear should be cleaned out to remove debris. The ear mites can be treated topically with any number of ear mite preparations licensed for use in cats, for at least 30 days. It is important to treat all other dogs and cats that have been in contact with the kittens. Ear mites are highly contagious, even to adult animals. Finally, it is very important to treat the hair coat of the kittens, especially the head and ear margins with a flea spray. Ear mite eggs are often laid on the hairs of the ear margins, and males migrate along the margins of the ear looking for females to breed. Using a flea control product on the body easily prevents reinfestation of the ears from mites migrating on the body.
iii. *Microsporum canis* and *Malassezia* spp. yeast can cause otic disease in kittens. *Demodex* spp. can also be found in the ears of kittens. Otic examinations, ear swab cytology, and mineral oil smears of ear exudate are the minimal diagnostics for cats or kittens presented with pruritic ears.

197 The inner pinna of a mixed breed dog is shown. Both inner pinnae are similar in appearance. The owner reports the dog developed small erythematous patches on the inner pinnae about 1 month ago. Since that time, the patches have become bilaterally symmetrical ulcerative lesions that are slowly enlarging (197). The dog is otherwise normal.

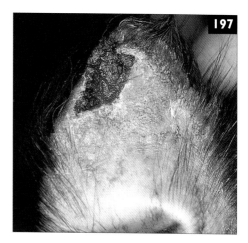

i. What are the differential diagnoses for these lesions?
ii. What diagnostic test is indicated?
iii. What is proliferative thrombo-vascular necrosis?

198 A 1-year-old male castrated orange tabby cat was presented for examination. of black spots in the mouth. The cat is healthy, and the spots are multifocal areas of black pigmentation on the cat's lips and gums (198).

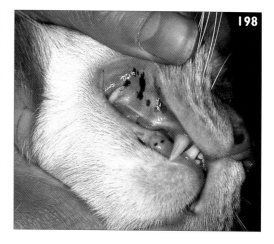

i. What is this condition called?
ii. How should this condition be treated?
iii. What is unique about this syndrome?

199 Lactophenol cotton blue stain is a 'vital stain'. This means it stains living cells although the cells die after contact with the stain. What is it used for?

197 i. The most likely differential diagnoses include drug eruptions, lupus erythematosus, vasculitis, thrombosis, ulcerations due to hyperadrenocorticism, and idiopathic proliferative thrombovascular necrosis of the pinnae.
ii. The most useful diagnostic test is a skin biopsy; a full thickness biopsy is necessary for diagnosis. Due to the location of the lesion and the technical difficulty involved in obtaining a sample from the ear pinnae, a wedge of tissue must be removed, as might be done in a cosmetic ear trim.
iii. Proliferative thrombovascular necrosis is a disease of unknown etiology with no age, breed, or sex predilection. Affected individuals develop small ulcers or erosions on the apical margin of the pinnae that spread along the concave surface. Eventually an elongated necrotic ulcer develops at the center of the lesion. The margins of the lesion may be thickened and scaly with a hyperpigmented margin. The lesions are often wedge shaped. As the lesion enlarges, necrosis occurs, and the ear margin becomes deformed (Scott *et al.*, 2001i). This was a case of proliferative thrombovascular necrosis of the pinnae. The patient responded to pentoxifylline therapy.

198 i. Lentigo, a very common hereditary pigmentary condition found in orange and yellow cats. Multifocal areas of black pigmentation on the gums, lips, and nose develop as the cat ages, and it is diagnosed based upon clinical signs.
ii. This is a cosmetic condition and does not require therapy.
iii. Lentigo simplex is unique because it is the only recognized inherited form of hypermelanosis in small animals.

199 This stain is used for the identification of fungal pathogens. The sticky side of clear acetate tape is pressed gently against the surface of a suspect colony (white or pale colony), and then placed over a drop of lactophenol cotton blue stain on a glass microscope slide. A second drop of stain is placed over the tape and a glass coverslip situated before microscopic examination. The macroconidia of *Microsporum canis* are shown (**199**). This slide was stained and 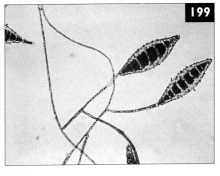 examined approximately 1 hour later. The lactophenol cotton blue stain was absorbed intracellularly making it easier to identify the macroconidia as those of *M. canis*. This stain is readily available through medical suppliers.

200 A 2-year-old golden retriever dog from the northern USA was presented for the problem of seasonal anal licking. The owners reported the dog had similar problems last year during the warm weather months. Careful questioning revealed that the symptoms were present during the warm months but tended to wax and wane every few weeks. The dog was otherwise healthy except for erythema on its paws. The owners couldn't agree as to whether or not the symptoms seen today were 'as bad as it gets, or not'. The owners took the dog home, decided to watch the lesions, keep a log of lesion severity, and note any changes in diet, or environment. Approximately 2 weeks later, the owners called and reported the dog's erythema had almost completely resolved but suddenly reappeared this morning. Yesterday they took the dog to an off-leash park for several

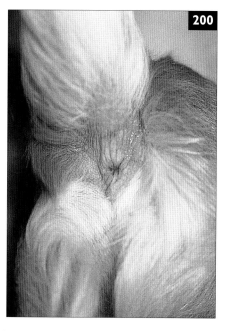

hours. Examination revealed severe erythema of the perineum, ventral inguinal region, and plantar surface of the paws (200).
i. What is the clinical diagnosis, and how can it be confirmed?
ii. The owners do not want to stop taking the dog to the park. What treatment options can the owners be offered? What other allergic disease could this dog be predisposed to?

201 Antihistamines are commonly used in veterinary dermatology as adjuvant therapy for the treatment of pruritus. Currently, both first and second generation antihistamines are used in clinical practice.
i. What is the primary mechanism of action of antihistamines?
ii. What is the primary difference between first and second generation antihistamines?
iii. What are the side-effects and adverse effects associated with the use of antihistamines?

200 i. An allergic contact reaction (type 4 hypersensitivity reaction/delayed reaction). In this case, it is important to confirm if the dog is having an allergic reaction to vegetation in the park. The dog should not be allowed to return to the park until all of the erythema resolves. Ideally, the dog should be examined to confirm this. Once the dog is normal, the owners should take the dog back to the same park under weather and temperature conditions similar to those on the day of the allergic reaction. The dog should be watched carefully for signs of anal pruritus and ventral erythema. If these develop within 24–72 hours after exposure to the park, a contact allergy is almost certain.

ii. It is possible this dog has a contact allergy to vegetation unique to this one park. The owners could wait until lesions resolve and then visit other parks to test this theory. It is also possible the dog has a contact reaction to vegetation that is common in the geographic region where they live. The most obvious solution to the problem is avoidance, but this is not always possible. Bathing the dog after it visits the park and pre-treatment with glucocorticoids are an option. Pentoxifylline (10 mg/kg q24h–q12h) has been used to treat dogs with contact allergies, and it may be reasonable to manage this dog's seasonal symptoms with this drug. The dog should be watched closely for development of clinical signs consistent with atopic dermatitis.

201 i. Antihistamines are classified as H1 and H2 receptor antagonists; the latter includes drugs such as cimetidine, ranitidine, and famotidine. Antihistamine drugs are considered competitive inhibitors and are most effective if used before histamine binds to receptor sites.

ii. Second generation antihistamines do not readily cross the blood–brain barrier. Therefore, they are associated with less sedation compared to first generation antihistamines. Second generation antihistamines also do not have antimuscarinic properties.

iii. Side-effects are unavoidable reactions associated with a drug's mechanism of action. Adverse effects are more severe and can be life threatening. The most common side-effects of first generation antihistamines are sedation and restlessness or excitement. These drugs can also cause antimuscarinic anticholinergic (atropine-like) side-effects. Animals may have a dry mouth leading to dental disease and halitosis. This may also lead to an increase in water consumption. Coughing due to a dry respiratory tract may also occur. Some animals become constipated or have diarrhea, have decreased appetite, and can develop abdominal bloating. Overdoses of second generation antihistamines can cause life-threatening cardiac episodes. These drugs should not be used concurrently with ketoconazole, itraconazole, or erythromycin or other drugs that are metabolized via the liver.

202 The external ear canal of a Chinese shar-pei dog is shown (202). Both ear canals appear similar. The owner reports the dog's hearing is diminished, and the dog has chronic ear infections. The external auditory canal is not visible.
i. What condition is being depicted here?
ii. What is the cause in this patient?
iii. What are the treatment options?

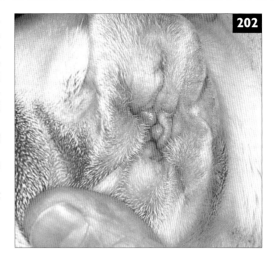

203 A female doberman pinscher dog was presented for the complaint of 'flank sucking' (203). The owner reported the skin in the flank area was chronically wet and the dog sucked, not nibbled, at the area.
i. What is 'flank sucking?'
ii. What diseases can mimic this disorder?

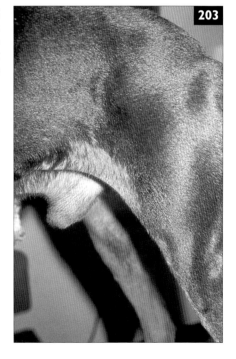

202 i. Stenotic ear canals.

ii. Stenosis of the ear canals occurs most commonly from inflammation and secondary fibrosis and calcification of the cartilaginous walls of the canal. In Chinese shar-pei dogs, the ear canal may be stenotic due to a conformational defect in which the ear canals are abnormally smaller and/or as a result of mucin deposition in the tissue, resulting in occlusion of the external ear canal. In some dogs, both conditions are present.

iii. Permanent resolution of stenotic ear canals in Chinese shar-pei dogs is not often possible since the underlying cause of the problem is usually a congenital malformation (narrowing of the ear canal) along with concurrent deposition of mucin. A lateral ear resection might provide relief to this patient; however, this does not usually resolve the problem because the healed surgical site is infiltrated with mucin and, over time, the surgical opening to the horizontal canal becomes occluded. The first thing to determine in this patient is whether or not there is a complicating bacterial or yeast infection. This may require sedation and careful sample collection using a microtip culture swab; the ear canal may be too occluded to pass a normal sized cotton tip applicator.

Second, skull radiographs or a CT scan will help determine the location, degree, and extent of the stenosis. In some dogs, the ear canal is of normal width, and the stenosis is located very distally (at the opening of the external meatus) in the vertical ear canal. In these patients, medical intervention (glucocorticoids) may be helpful. If the canal is uniformly small (vertical and horizontal canal), medical management of the stenosis tends not to be beneficial. Surgical treatments (i.e. lateral ear resections) are often unsuccessful in this breed for the reasons mentioned above. Systemic glucocorticoids (1–2 mg/kg PO q24h) for 10–30 days will often decrease mucin production and provide some relief of the stenosis. This relief is temporary, but it is often the only option available.

203 i. Flank sucking is currently believed to be a type of psychomotor epilepsy. It is similar to tail sucking in cats. Flank sucking can occur in any breed of dog but is particularly common in doberman pinschers.

ii. Any skin disease that affects the flanks of dogs and causes discomfort must be ruled out prior to making this diagnosis. Clinical signs of hair loss, erythema, hyperpigmentation, lichenification, inflammation, nibbling or chewing, and salivary staining, should be considered evidence that there is an underlying skin disease causing the behavior. Skin biopsies should also be performed prior to making this diagnosis. Any evidence of inflammation suggests an organic disease. Flank sucking may respond to anticonvulsant therapy (e.g. phenobarbital), and response to glucocorticoids is evidence that there is an organic pruritic cause.

204 The owner reports that for the last 3 years, this 6-year-old male boxer dog has had recurrent hair loss every winter over the dorsum and the lumbosacral area (204). The hair coat regrows in the spring, but by fall, the alopecic pattern shown starts to develop. Skin scrapings and dermatophyte cultures are consistently negative. Thyroid function tests, low-dose dexamethasone suppression test, ACTH stimulation test, and adrenal panel are normal. The lesions do not respond to oral antibiotics, and the owner practices flea control. The dog is not pruritic.

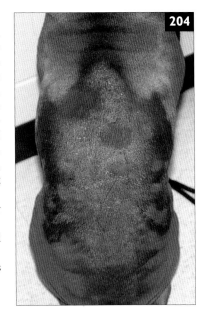

i. What is the most likely diagnosis or diagnoses?
ii. What is the cause of this syndrome, and how is it treated?
iii. What histological findings characterize this disease?

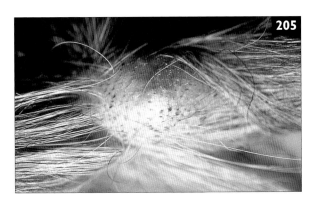

205 The owner of a golden retriever dog reported a focal area of scaling and hair loss on the proximal third of her dog's tail. Over the last year, the area has become increasingly more alopecic, swollen, and 'dotted'. After closer examination, it is noted that the 'dotting' is caused by follicular plugging and comedones (205).
i. This is a common lesion in older dogs. What is this condition called, and what treatment is needed?
ii. What skin diseases can occur at this site?
iii. What is this lesion's origin?

204 i. Seasonal flank alopecia. Despite the name, there is no consistent season for the hair loss. Some dogs lose their hair in the spring and summer and regrow it in the fall and winter, while in other dogs the reverse pattern occurs.

ii. The etiology of seasonal flank alopecia is unknown. It may be due to seasonal variations in hormones, particularly melatonin; however, this has not been proven. Because some dogs will have only one episode while others will develop this condition year after year, the prognosis is unpredictable. Anecdotally, some dogs have responded to subcutaneous implantation of melatonin (3×12 mg SC implants), while others responded to oral melatonin (3–6 mg q8h). Response was slow, and improvement may have been coincidental. These dogs have normal endocrine function tests.

iii. Compatible histological findings include follicular atrophy and infundibular hyperkeratosis. Hair follicles are dysplastic and are described as being octopus- or jellyfish-like in appearance (Miller and Dunstan, 1993).

205 i. Oval tail gland hyperplasia. This lesion may occur in all dogs but is most noticeable in intact male dogs. The glands of this region are testosterone sensitive, explaining why they are more likely to be problematic in intact male dogs.

ii. In dogs with primary or secondary seborrhea or increased concentrations of androgens, the glandular tissue hypertrophies. When this occurs, the gland enlarges, the primary hairs are lost, and the area becomes scaly and/or greasy. In some cases, the gland may become infected. In addition, skin tumors (adenomas and adeno-carcinomas) may develop at this site. In most cases, hair loss and comedones require no treatment and are considered cosmetic defects. If the gland becomes infected, it should be treated as an area of local deep pyoderma. The area should be hot packed, lanced if necessary, and systemic antibiotic therapy administered for 21–30 days. These lesions tend to recur, and castration may be helpful if the dog is intact.

iii. The oval tail gland (tail gland, preen gland, supracaudal gland) is a specialized skin gland found in all wild Canidae and in dogs. It is comprised of simple hairs and numerous large sebaceous and circumanal glands, starts at the fifth to seventh coccygeal vertebra, and can extend the entire length of the tail. It is clinically visible in most dogs. The function of the gland is unknown, but it is believed to be involved in olfactory species recognition in canines. Histologically, the gland is comprised of hepatoid cells. These glandular structures empty directly into hair follicles.

206 A 5-year-old dachshund dog is presented for pruritus, hair loss, and crusting of 4 months' duration (206a, b). Skin scrapings and dermatophyte cultures are negative, but impression smears reveal large numbers of cocci and smaller numbers of *Malassezia* organisms. The dog's clinical signs do not improve after 4 weeks of cephalexin and keto-conazole treatment. The dog is also treated for scabies, and the owners practice flea control. At the time of presentation, the dog is depressed and febrile. The owner reports the crusting lesions tend to wax and wane, and the dog becomes depressed approximately 24 hours before new lesions develop. Clinical examination reveals large flaccid pustules spanning several hair follicles, and there is a slight greenish tinge to the pustules.

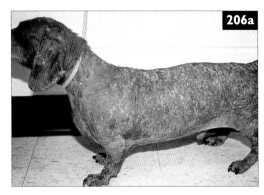

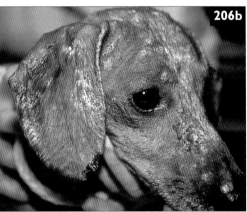

i. What are the dog's dermatological problems?
ii. What is the most likely differential diagnosis, and what diagnostic test(s) are needed to confirm it?
iii. Is there any in-house diagnostic test available to make a presumptive diagnosis pending confirmation?

207 Cyclophosphamide, chlorambucil, azathioprine, and chrysotherapy are commonly used to treat immune-mediated skin diseases.
i. What is the mechanism of action of these drugs and what are the most common adverse effects?
ii. Which of these drugs is contraindicated in cats?

206 i. Pruritus and pustular eruption. If intact pustules were not found, crusting would have been an appropriate problem to pursue. The major causes of pruritus were ruled out by previous diagnostics or treatments, and the clinical signs are inconsistent with allergic skin disease. Therefore, the pustular eruptions should be considered the primary problem. The pruritus is most likely the result of inflammation associated with the underlying disease.

ii. The most likely diagnosis is PF. Multiple skin biopsies for routine histopathological examination should be taken, and collection should occur immediately because intact primary lesions (pustules) are very transient and fragile. Since the pustules span several hair follicles, a 6–8 mm skin biopsy instrument will be needed. Submission of intact pustules is critical, so the skin should not be scrubbed or wiped before specimen collection. Alternatively, an elliptical incision using a scalpel blade can be used to collect a specimen. It is important to mount the material on a piece of a wooden tongue depressor subcutaneous side down prior to putting the specimen in formalin. A bacterial culture of the contents of an intact pustule should also be submitted to rule out the rare possibility that this is a cephalexin resistant bacterial pyoderma.

iii. Since this patient is presenting with a wave of pustules, impression smears of pustular contents can be made. Rafts of acanthocytes (noncornified epithelial cells) amid a sea of neutrophils are often seen in cases of PF. It is also helpful to look for the presence of bacteria. This was a case of canine PF.

207 i. Cyclophosphamide is an alkylating agent that inhibits mitosis by interfering with DNA replication and RNA transcription and replication. The major toxic side-effects include hemorrhagic cystitis, bladder fibrosis, teratogenesis, infertility, alopecia, nausea, bone marrow depression, and increased susceptibility to infections. Chlorambucil is another alkylating agent that cross links DNA. It is slow acting and less toxic than cyclophosphamide. The most common adverse effects include bone marrow suppression, anorexia, vomiting, and diarrhea. Alopecia and delayed hair growth can occur. Azathioprine is a synthetic 6-mercaptopurine that is metabolized in the liver to 6-mercaptopurine and other active metabolites. This drug antagonizes purine metabolism and interferes with DNA and RNA synthesis. The most common adverse effects include bone marrow suppression, vomiting, pancreatitis, alopecia, and diarrhea. The mechanism of action of chrysotherapy (gold salts) is unknown. It is available in two forms oral (auranofin 29%) and aurothioglucose (50% gold). Gold salts have anti-inflammatory and immunomodulating activity with a delayed onset of action. The most common adverse effects are skin rashes, proteinuria, and bone marrow suppression.

ii. Azathioprine should not be used in cats because it can cause fatal leucopenia and thrombocytopenia.

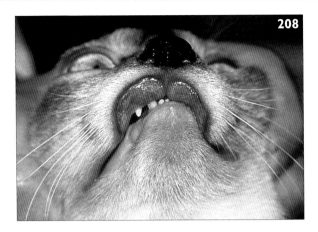

208 A Siamese cat was presented for a lesion on its lip (208). This type of lesion is very common in cats.
i. What is the clinical diagnosis?
ii. What are the treatment options?

209 A 7-year-old male collie dog with nasal depigmentation and crusting on the dorsum of the nose for the last 6 years is shown (209). Lesions are worse during the summer and almost completely resolve during the winter. The owners presented the dog for examination because the lesions have not resolved this winter. The nose is proliferative and deformed, and the dog has intermittent nasal bleeding.
i. The waxing and waning lesions are initially most suggestive of which disease?
ii. Given that the lesions have worsened over time and are no longer resolving, what is the working diagnosis now?
iii. The owners declined a skin biopsy, but would like medical management. How should the dog be treated given the limited information available?

208 i. Eosinophilic ulcer or indolent ulcer. This is a reaction pattern lesion in cats, and it may occur bilaterally or unilaterally. Cats with these lesions frequently have eosinophilic granulomas and/or eosinophilic plaques. These lesions may or may not be recurrent after initial treatment. If recurrent, underling allergic diseases (FAD, food allergy, and/or atopy) should be investigated. Unilateral lesions on the upper lip are common at the site of a previous dermatophyte infection, and focal inflammation or trauma may be triggers for unilateral lesions as well.

ii. The lesions may resolve spontaneously, especially those that are small and unilateral. Large unilateral or bilateral lesions should be treated because they can rapidly enlarge and become disfiguring. Methylprednisone acetate (20 mg/cat SC) every 2 weeks until the lesions resolve (4–6 weeks) is effective. Although oral prednisone (2.2–4.4 mg/kg) is also effective, many cats do not seem to respond to oral medications as well as they do to parenteral therapy. This is most likely due to the difficulty encountered by owners when orally medicating cats. Progestational compounds are not recommended due to the risk of development of diabetes mellitus and adrenal suppression. Surgical excision or laser therapy is not necessary except in rare refractory cases, which are often due to an undiagnosed allergic disease.

209 i. The symptoms are most suggestive of nasal solar dermatitis or 'collie nose'. Collie nose was a name given to a waxing and waning skin disease of the dorsal nose and nasal planum of collies and Shetland sheepdogs, exacerbated by sun exposure.

ii. Cutaneous lupus erythematosus. It is common for cutaneous lupus erythematosus to wax and wane over time and gradually worsen, especially if left untreated, or if no effort is made to minimize solar-induced relapses.

iii. The owner's decision not to allow a skin biopsy to confirm the diagnosis is unfortunate. Although the most likely diagnosis is cutaneous lupus erythematosus, the deformity of the nose is worrisome, and it is possible this dog has developed a squamous cell carcinoma. This tumor is common in chronic cases of cutaneous lupus erythematosus. In addition, cutaneous lymphoma can masquerade as cutaneous lupus erythematosus. If a definitive diagnosis of cutaneous lupus erythematosus were known, this dog would be a good candidate for aggressive immunosuppressive therapy with glucocorticoids and/or azathioprine to induce the lesions into remission. Once the lesions are in remission, potent topical glucocorticoids and sunscreens could be used to minimize relapses and control active lesions. In this patient, oral vitamin E therapy, tetracycline and niacinamide, topical fluorinated glucocorticoids, and sunscreens would be recommended. The cost of systemic immunosuppressive therapy and monitoring would far exceed that of a skin biopsy procedure and histopathology. Cost constraints do not justify forgoing a skin biopsy.

210 Raised white lesions are shown on the head of a cat (210). Similar lesions are present elsewhere on the body, and some of these lesions have ulcerated. The lesions developed approximately 6 months ago, and the cat was recently diagnosed with diabetes mellitus. Skin biopsy findings revealed a nodular to diffuse infiltrate of macrophages, and multinucleated histiocytic giant cells.

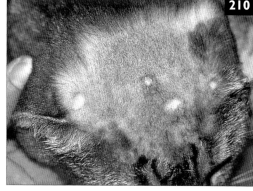

i. What is the most likely diagnosis based upon the information provided?
ii. What is the treatment of choice?

211 A middle-aged dog was presented for evaluation of its ventral abdomen. Note the multifocal, raised, fluctuant nodules (211). The owner reported the lesions developed rapidly, ruptured, and drained an oily, yellow-brown material. The lesions were painful upon palpation, and the dog was depressed, febrile, and had generalized lymphadenopathy. Additional historical and physical examination findings include depression,

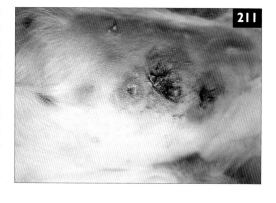

fever, anorexia, pain upon palpation of the abdomen, and vomiting.
i. What are the differential diagnoses? The oily yellow-brown discharge is consistent with which differential diagnoses?
ii. How should skin biopsy specimens be collected for histopathology?
iii. What is the pathogenesis of this condition, and what metabolic diseases can lead to these lesions?

212 Chlorhexidine solution (8 oz [240 ml]) of 0.05% is to be dispensed for wound flushing. The stock solution is 2%. How is this prescription compounded?

210 i. Xanthomatosis. This is a benign granulomatous skin disease resulting from abnormalities in lipid metabolism. It is most commonly seen in cats with idiopathic hyperlipidemia or diabetes mellitus due to naturally occurring causes or drugs (i.e. glucocorticoids, megestrol acetate).
ii. Lesions associated with diabetes mellitus will spontaneously resolve with appropriate treatment for the diabetes mellitus. If the lesions are due to drugs, they will resolve once the drug is discontinued.

211 i. Deep pyoderma, cutaneous cysts, neoplasia, infections, panniculitis, and foreign body reaction. The oily yellow-brown discharge is the result of fat necrosis due to inflammation of subcutaneous fat, and the most likely diagnosis here is panniculitis.
ii. A deep wedge biopsy specimen or an excisional nodular biopsy using cold steel is recommended. Special stains for microorganisms and examination of the specimen under polarized light for foreign bodies should be requested.
iii. The lipocyte is a relatively fragile cell that is vulnerable to trauma, ischemia, and inflammatory diseases. Upon injury or death, lipid is released that is degraded into glycerol and fatty acids. The latter are very inflammatory and start a cycle of inflammation and further cell death. The free lipids and marked inflammatory reaction result in a granulomatous tissue reaction. Panniculitis has been associated with a number of metabolic diseases. Pancreatitis has been diagnosed in dogs with necrotizing steatitis and concurrent gastrointestinal symptoms. Most cases of nodular panniculitis are idiopathic in origin.

212 First convert both strengths from % to mg/ml:
Available: 2% = 2 g/100 ml = 2000 mg/100 ml = 20 mg/ml
Needed: 0.05% = 0.05 g/100 ml = 50 mg/100 ml = 0.5 mg/ml

Then, calculate the number of mg of chlorhexidine needed in 240 ml of solution:
0.5 mg/ml × 240 ml = 120 mg

Next, calculate how many ml of chlorhexidine 2% (20 mg/ml) is needed to get that amount:
120 mg ÷ 20 mg/ml = 6 ml

Then, calculate the quantity of distilled water to add to get a 240 ml solution of chlorhexidine 0.05%:
240 ml – 6 ml = 234 ml of distilled water

Therefore, 6 ml of 2% chlorhexidine solution would be diluted in 234 ml of distilled water to obtain 240 ml (8 oz) of 0.05% chlorhexidine solution.

213 A dog is presented by the owners for examination because it 'yelps' when petted on or near the ears. They also report that he has stopped chewing on his toys and refuses to eat hard food. The dog is irritable and doesn't want to play. These symptoms have been present intermittently for over 4 months. The ear is erythematous, exudative, and malodorous (213a). The dog has been treated several times for otitis externa with various topical ear flushes and topical ear medications. Upon physical examination, it is difficult to examine the ears without causing pain to the patient. There is an odorous creamy brown exudate present. Cytological examination of the exudate is shown (213b, c). The dog resists having its mouth opened.

i. What is the working diagnosis, and what diagnostics should be performed?
ii. Pending the results, what is the treatment plan?
iii. What is the long-term treatment plan?

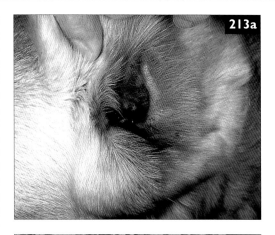

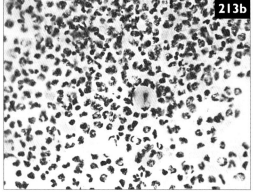

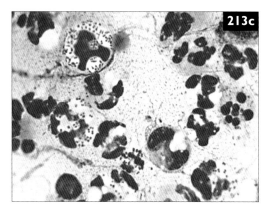

213: Answer

213 i. The working diagnoses are otitis externa and otitis media. The pain upon examination and manipulation of the ear canal is consistent with both otitis externa and otitis media. The reluctance to chew on hard toys or food and to have its mouth opened is compatible with pain at the temporomandibular joint or region. These symptoms are common in dogs with otitis media, but not in dogs with otitis externa. Finally, the cytological preparations show septic inflammation with bacteria (cocci and rods). Similar cytological findings could be found in patients with otitis externa, but in this case, the clinical signs and duration of the otitis are more compatible with otitis media. At this visit, a bacterial culture and sensitivity should be done as it is important to determine which microbial organisms are present. Yeast may be present but not seen on the cytological preparation due to the amount of exudates.

ii. Pending the culture and sensitivity, treat with systemic antibiotics (ciprofloxacin 20 mg/kg PO q24h) because *Pseudomonas* is suspected as the cause of the otitis media. Topical ear preparations will be ineffective in this patient for several reasons. First, these products are rarely efficacious in the presence of purulent exudates. Second, owners are often unable to medicate adequately dogs with painful ears. Finally, therapeutic concentrations of antimicrobials in ear canal tissue and/or in the middle ear cannot be achieved with most commercially available topical drugs. In addition to the systemic antimicrobial therapy, oral prednisone was prescribed for both its analgesic and anti-inflammatory effects since much of the pain in these patients is due to swelling of ear tissue. Furthermore, the ear canal epithelium and lining of the tympanic bulla is very secretory and glucocorticoid therapy helps to diminish the secretions. The owners reported the dog's attitude and appetite improved within 48 hours of starting therapy.

iii. This dog has a history of recurrent otitis externa, and the most common cause of this is an undiagnosed otitis media. The ear should be reexamined every 3–4 weeks via otoscopic examination, cytological examination, and ear culture. The end point of treatment is a negative ear culture. The dog will also require frequent and careful ear cleaning. Depending upon the severity of the infection, a middle ear irrigation to remove debris from the tympanic bullae may be needed. This is often necessary in cases of *Pseudomonas* ear infections and is performed under general anesthesia. Ear cleaning could be done at the first visit or 2–3 days after systemic initiation of antimicrobial therapy.

214 A purebred 2-year-old female vizsla dog was presented for the complaint of hair loss. Note the multifocal circular areas (**214a**). Close examination of the skin revealed fine white scales and hair casts. Previous diagnostics and treatments included skins scrapings, impression smears, fungal cultures, flea control, and 30 days of oral cephalexin (30 mg/kg PO q12h). There was no response to treatment, and all previous diagnostic testing was negative. A skin biopsy was performed, and a photomicrograph of the specimen is shown. Note the accumulation of inflammatory cells at the level of the sebaceous gland (**214b**).

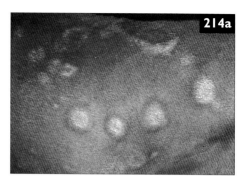

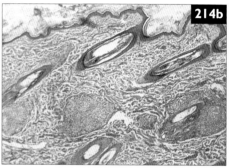

i. What is the diagnosis?
ii. What are the recommendations for breeding and treatment?
iii. What is the pathogenesis of this disorder?

215 *Pythium insidiosum* and *Lagenidium* spp. are aquatic oomycetes that cause systemic and dermatological disease in dogs living in the south-eastern USA. Dogs with dermatological lesions are often presented for the problem of nonhealing wounds. Diagnosis is made via history, clinical signs, culture of the organism (if possible), and histological findings. Unfortunately, it if often difficult to distinguish between the histological findings caused by lagenidiosis and zygomycosis making diagnosis difficult. Recently, a *Pythium insidiosum*- and *Lagenidium*-specific PCR assay was described to detect the oomycete DNA in animal tissues (Znajda *et al.*, 2002). This assay is to be tested on several samples from infected dogs. Primers specific for *P. insidiosum* (322 bp product) and the canine pathogenic *Lagenidium* species (266 bp product) are provided. The samples arrive labeled 1–6, but no other information is provided other than one of the samples is from an uninfected dog and is to be used as a control. No further information is needed; the PCR reaction can be run and the results analyzed using a 1% agarose gel containing EB.

i. What is expected to be seen on the gel?
ii. How would it be determined that one of the samples was indeed the control, and the results observed on the agarose gel are not simply because the PCR reaction failed to work?

214 i. Granulomatous sebaceous adenitis.

ii. Breeding from affected dogs should be avoided because of the possible hereditary nature of this disease. There is no effective, or predictable treatment for this disorder, and care should be taken to monitor dogs for the development of secondary bacterial and/or yeast infections.

iii. The pathogenesis of this disease is unknown but may include an inherited and/or developmental defect in sebaceous glands, a cell-mediated immune attack on sebaceous glands, or a defect in keratinization. In some breeds (e.g. standard poodles), there is evidence of an autosomal recessive mode of inheritance. There is a breed predilection for standard poodles, akitas, vizslas, samoyeds, and Belgian sheepdogs.

215 i. A product of 322 bp, indicating *P. insidiosum*, or a 266 bp product, indicating the canine pathogenic *Lagenidium* spp should be present. No product would be expected from the control sample. A representative gel is shown (**215**). Note that molecular weight markers must also be loaded on the gel in order to identify the size of the products. The markers used are 100–1000 bp in size and increase 100 bp for each marker. Lanes 1, 2, and 5 indicate *P. insidiosum* infection, lanes 3 and 6 indicate canine pathogenic *Lagenidium* spp., lane 4 is the control (no band present), and lane 7 contains the molecular weight markers.

ii. Because a band is not present in lane 4, the PCR reaction may have failed for this sample. However, a band would not be expected in one of the lanes since it is known that one sample is the control. An easy way to verify that the reaction worked, and that the sample was indeed from an uninfected dog is to run a separate PCR assay for a gene made by all animal cells, such as the genes encoding the protein β-actin or GAPDH, an enzyme found in the glycolytic pathway and thus present in all animal tissues. If primers for GAPDH are provided that generate a 300 bp product, a PCR assay for all six samples should be run, using these primers. If a product of 300 bp is present in all the samples this indicates that sample 4 contained intact DNA that could be used for a PCR reaction, and the lack of a band in the experimental gel lane 4 was because the dog was not infected.

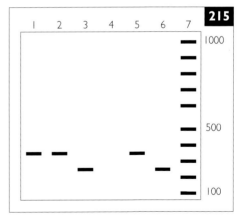

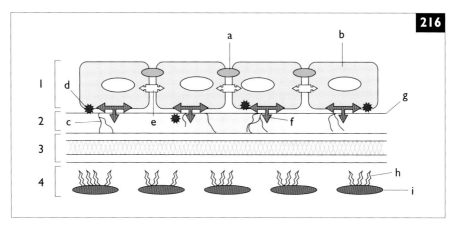

216 A diagrammatic representation of the DEJ is shown (216).
i. What is the purpose of the basement membrane zone?
ii. Identify the four major regions of the epidermis (1–4).
iii. Identify each of the components of the DEJ (a–i).

217 A middle-aged cat was treated with repeated subcutaneous injections of methylprednisone acetate for chronic asthma. The owner reported the hair on the lateral thorax, which was clipped 6 months ago for an ultrasound evaluation, has not regrown (217). A skin biopsy of the area is 'compatible with an endocrine alopecia'. What is the most likely diagnosis of the lack of hair regrowth?

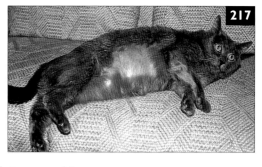

218 Canine demodicosis has three clinical presentations. What are they and how are they characterized?

216 i. The basement membrane zone is important because it anchors the epidermis to the dermis, maintains a normal and functional epidermis, maintains tissue architecture, helps in wound healing, functions as a barrier, and regulates the transport of nutrition between the epidermis and dermis.

ii. Basal layer (1), lamina lucida (2), lamina densa (3), and sublamina densa (4).

iii. The components are as follows: adherens junction (a), basal cell (b), anchoring filaments (c), focal adhesion (d), desmosome (e), hemidesmosome (f), basal plasma membrane (g), anchoring fibrils (h), anchoring plaques (i).

217 Iatrogenic feline hyperadrenocorticism. Exogenous administration of glucocorticoids can cause slow hair regrowth in both dogs and cats. Compared to dogs, owners of cats report fewer adverse effects of exogenous glucocorticoid administration. It may be that cats have fewer problems or the common adverse effects (i.e. polyuria, polydipsia, and polyphagia) are less noticeable in house cats. Long-term administration of glucocorticoids in cats can cause clinical signs similar to naturally occurring feline hyperadrenocorticism, including muscle wasting, hair loss, thin hypotonic skin, easy bruising, spontaneous tears of the skin, and mild seborrhea.

Unlike dogs, cats rarely show signs of polyuria and polydipsia from glucocorticoid administration. Diabetes mellitus is common secondary to chronic glucocorticoid administration in cats, and this disease is the primary cause of polyuria and polydipsia. One unique clinical feature of iatrogenic disease in cats is medial curling of the ear pinnae, an element not been seen in naturally occurring disease. This cat regrew his hair coat approximately 1 year after the glucocorticoids were discontinued. Focal areas of hair loss at the site of glucocorticoid injections can occur in cats, and owners should be warned of this complication. If this cosmetic risk is a concern to the owners, the injection can be administered in the inguinal region.

218 Localized, generalized, and adult-onset demodicosis. Localized demodicosis is characterized by one or more focal areas of hair loss in which mites are found on deep skin scrapings. Mites are not found in normal adjacent skin. Approximately 90% of these cases will resolve without treatment. Generalized demodicosis is characterized by the finding of *Demodex* mites on skin scrapings in both affected and normal appearing skin. Only 50% of dogs with generalized demodicosis will be cured with therapy. Adult-onset demodicosis is characterized by the development of demodicosis in an older dog with no known prior history of demodicosis. Adult-onset demodicosis is believed to develop as a result of an underlying systemic disorder, e.g. diabetes mellitus, neoplasia, or excessive glucocorticoid administration. If the underlying disease is treated, adult-onset demodicosis will often resolve.

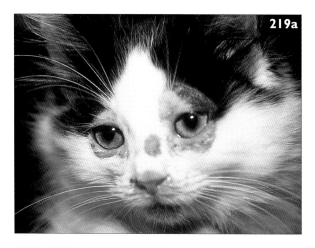

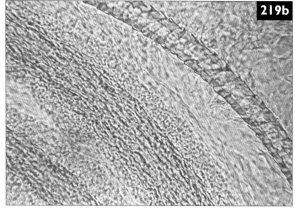

219 A kitten was presented for hair loss and erythema on the face (**219a**). The kitten was obtained from a farm. A Wood's lamp evaluation was positive, and several hairs were plucked and examined under potassium hydroxide (KOH). A preparation of a normal hair and an abnormal hair that was Wood's lamp-positive is shown (**219b**).

i. What is a Wood's lamp, what is it used for, what are the limitations, and what is the possible interpretation of the positive Wood's lamp evaluation?

ii. What is the possible interpretation of the KOH preparation, and can a definitive diagnosis be made at this time?

iii. What advantage would there be using a killed *Microsporum canis* vaccine in this patient?

219 i. A Wood's light is a hand-held lamp that emits long-wave ultraviolet radiation through a nickel or cobalt glass filter (Moriello, 2001). The filter is opaque to all light except for a band between 320 and 400 nm. Fluorescence occurs when shorter wavelengths of light (340–400 nm) emitted by the Wood's light are absorbed, and radiation of longer wavelengths (visible light) are emitted. The Wood's lamp is not very helpful in the diagnosis of dermatophytosis in small animals because it is only a screening tool. False positives can occur from ointments, shampoos, and misinterpretations. A true positive is apple green in color, and many people mistake the yellow-green of oily seborrhea as positive, or the blue white of dust as positive. In addition, it is very important to note that many fibers, especially carpet fibers will glow bright green when exposed to a Wood's lamp. The lamp needs to be warmed up for 5–10 minutes prior to use to stabilize the wavelength. Furthermore, the examination should take at least 5 minutes in a darkened room, allowing a clinician's eyes to adapt and see the fluorescence. In this case, the Wood's lamp examination is suggestive of a possible dermatophyte infection. The only organism of veterinary importance that fluoresces is *Microsporum canis*; however, <50% of strains are detected by this method. If apple green glowing hairs are found, they can be sampled for culture and/or direct examination with KOH.

ii. Clearing agents cause the material in the background to swell and become somewhat opaque, leaving keratinized hairs and spores more refractile. The microscope condenser should be low along with the lamp light intensity. From a 10x magnification, infected versus noninfected hairs can be seen. This KOH preparation shows a normal hair and two infected hairs. The infected hairs are wider, more filamentous, and large numbers of ectothrix spores can be seen in a cuff surrounding the hairs. These results allow a diagnosis of dermatophytosis to be made in this kitten, specifically *M. canis* dermatophytosis.

iii. Topical therapy alone with lime sulfur or enilconazole is an effective therapy. Lufenuron is ineffective in the treatment of dermatophytosis and as a possible preventative, thus, it is not recommended. Killed *M. canis* vaccines have been approved as an adjuvant therapy in the treatment of dermatophytosis. The vaccine alone will not cure a clinical case of dermatophytosis. It will, however, induce an immune response in the cat resulting in a temporary lessening of clinical signs. Presumably, this will decrease the severity of the lesions and may lessen shedding of infective hairs and spores into the environment.

220 An adult dog was presented for examination of its mucocutaneous junction and oral mucosa. The owner reported the dog was depressed, anorexic, drooling, and had a strong odor emanating from its mouth. Note the ulcerations and erosions (220a, b). These lesions did not respond to a course of oral antibiotics, and similar lesions are present on the prepuce and anus. Intact vesicles were found on the borders of these lesions. Except for the

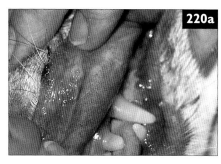

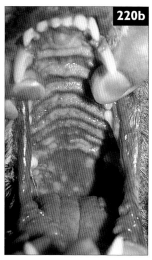

skin lesions, no other abnormalities were found on physical examination. A complete blood count revealed a leukocytosis and a stress leukogram. A serum chemistry panel, urinalysis, ANA, and skin scraping were normal or negative. Impression smears of the lesions showed neutrophils and cellular debris, but fungal organisms were not found. Skin biopsy findings report suprabasilar acantholysis with cleft and vesicle formation. Basal epidermal cells in a row of 'tombstones' were attached to the basement membrane zone. Minimal dermal inflammation was seen. DIF testing revealed intercellular fluorescence, and special stains were negative for yeast or bacteria.

i. What are the major differential diagnoses for oral and mucocutaneous ulcerations?

ii. Based upon the clinical signs and biopsy findings, what is the most likely diagnosis and why?

221 Scaling can be noted on the dog's hair coat shown (221). Clinical examination reveals bacterial pyoderma and fleas. The scaling resolves with treatment of the bacterial pyoderma and fleas.

i. The 'scales' are also referred as seborrhea. What is the difference between primary and secondary seborrhea? What type does this patient have?

ii. What are keratolytic and keratoplastic agents?

iii. What is the mechanism of action of tar, sulfur, and salicylic acid?

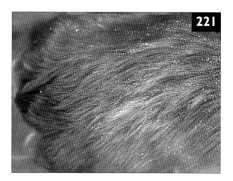

220 i. The major differential diagnoses include SLE, BP, erythema multiforme, pemphigus vulgaris, drug reactions, candidiasis, and cutaneous lymphoma.
ii. The most likely diagnosis is pemphigus vulgaris. The skin biopsy findings are incompatible with the other differential diagnoses except cutaneous drug reaction, which can mimic almost any known skin disease. The presence of acantholytic cells is typical of the pemphigus complex. The differentiation of the pemphigus group is based upon clinical signs, and the location of clefting and acantholysis in the epidermis. Pemphigus foliaceus/erythematosus are characterized by diffuse scaling and crusting and acantholysis in the intragranular layer (high in the epidermis). Pemphigus vulgaris is characterized by mucocutaneous ulceration and clefting and acantholysis in the deep epidermis. The description of the 'row of tombstones' (i.e. basal cells just below the cleft) is a classic descriptive finding compatible with pemphigus vulgaris. DIF in pemphigus is intercellular but is not always positive. It should not be done in lieu of routine histopathology, and the diagnosis should not be discarded because it is negative. This was a case of pemphigus vulgaris.

221 i. The general term for scaling is called 'seborrhea'. This is not a clinical diagnosis, but rather a clinical description of a type of skin lesion. Seborrhea has two basic etiologies: primary seborrhea and secondary seborrhea. Primary seborrhea is caused by an inherited disorder of keratinization of the epidermis. This disorder is common in many breeds of dogs including West Highland white terriers, cocker spaniels, and German shepherd dogs. It is a chronic disorder and diagnosis is made by ruling out all other possible causes. Secondary seborrhea occurs when any external or internal disease alters the normal development of the skin. It is simply the skin's response to insult. It may occur as a result of inflammation, infection, self-trauma, and poor nutrition. In clinical practice, some of the most common causes of secondary seborrhea are bacterial pyoderma, fleas, and *Cheyletiella* infestations. This patient had secondary seborrhea.
ii. A keratolytic agent facilitates decreased cohesion between keratinocytes, desquamation, and shedding. This results in a softening of the stratum corneum and removal of scales. A keratoplastic agent attempts to normalize the process of keratinization.
iii. Tar is keratolytic, keratoplastic, and mildly degreasing. It is believed to normalize the process of keratinization by decreasing DNA production, with a resultant decrease in the mitotic index of basal cells. Sulfur is keratolytic and keratoplastic, probably through the interaction of sulfur with cysteine in keratinocytes. Salicylic acid is keratoplastic.

222 The nose of the dog shown (222) depicts a common syndrome seen in Siberian husky, golden retriever, Labrador retriever, and Bernese mountain dogs. It can be very distressing to owners.

i. What is the clinical name for this syndrome, what is the lay person's common name for this change?

ii. What is poliosis, and what disease has it been associated with?

iii. In what breed of cat has periocular leukotrichia been documented, and what factors are associated with its development?

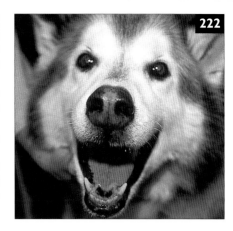

223 A 9-year-old female Siamese cat is presented early one morning by an overwrought owner for the complaint of 'its skin pulled off'. The owner was dragging the cat out from under the bed when the cat's skin literally ripped off in her hand. There was minimal bleeding associated with the episode, and the cat did not appear to be in any discomfort. Physical examination was normal, except for the skin, which was extremely fragile. Full thickness tears were produced with only minor trauma to the skin (223a, b).

i. What is this cat's dermatological problem?

ii. What are the differential diagnoses?

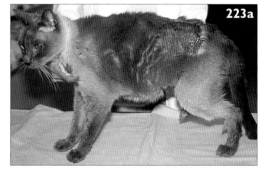

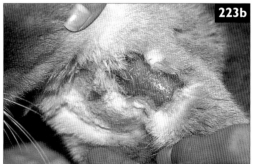

224 What is phaeohyphomycosis?

222 i. Nasal hypopigmentation. Owners frequently refer to this syndrome as 'snow nose'. It is characterized by a strip of depigmentation down the center of the nose. In some breeds, e.g. Labrador retrievers, the nose may turn from black to brown instead. There is no treatment for this condition, and affected dogs do not seem to be bothered by it. The cause is unknown and may be genetic as it is often seen in related littermates. The depigmentation can be seasonal (i.e. winter), and some noses will spontaneously repigment in the summer, hence the name 'snow nose'.
ii. Poliosis is a premature graying of the hair or skin, and it has been associated with canine uveodermatologic syndrome.
iii. Periocular leukotrichia has been diagnosed most commonly in Siamese cats, usually females. Affected cats develop lightening of the hair around the eyes, and they look like they have a white mask. The condition is transient, and normal coat color usually returns within 1–3 cycles. It can be associated with pregnancy, dietary deficiencies, and systemic illnesses.

223 i. Skin fragility or acquired feline skin fragility syndrome. Feline skin fragility syndrome is a term used to describe easily torn, damaged, thin skin that is damaged with little or no trauma. The skin may be translucent, and there may be concurrent partial alopecia. The skin is not hyperextensible as is seen in collagen disorders such as cutaneous asthenia. This syndrome should be considered a dermatological manifestation of systemic disease.
ii. Fragile full thickness tears in the skin of cats can occur with cutaneous asthenia, pancreatic neoplasia, liver disease (hepatic lipidosis, cholangiohepatitis, or cholangiocarcinoma), progesterone administration, iatrogenic and naturally occurring hyperadrenocorticism, phenytoin administration, and nephrosis. In some cats, no underlying abnormality is found. This patient had naturally occurring feline hyperadrenocorticism. If the underlying metabolic disease can be treated, the cat will regain normal skin integrity.

224 This is a subcutaneous infection of the skin caused by traumatic inoculation of saprophytes. These lesions can be clinically indistinguishable from mycetomas, tumors, or abscesses. They are diagnosed via histological examination of tissue, and the hallmark findings are pigmented, septate, branched or unbranched hyphae. Tissue granules are not a feature of this fungal disease. Treatment is difficult and surgical excision of the lesion is the treatment of choice but recurrence is common. Commonly isolated fungi include *Bipolaris spiceferum* (*Drechslera* spp.), *Phialemonium*, *Pseudomicrodochium* and *Xylahypha* (*Cladosporium* spp.).

225 The owners of a 3-year-old dog presented it on emergency because it was depressed and showed pain when touched (225). The dog had acutely developed anorexia, lethargy, and depression over the last 24 hours. Upon physical examination the dog was febrile and had generalized erythema of the skin. Because touching the skin was very painful for the dog during the examination, a thorough exam was difficult, and the dog needed to be sedated. After sedation, oral ulcerations and cutaneous bullae were found on the skin. Skin biopsies were obtained at this time, and the dog was treated symptomatically with fluid and electrolyte therapy. The hair coat was clipped and topical silver sulfadiazine was applied to the lesions to manage sepsis.

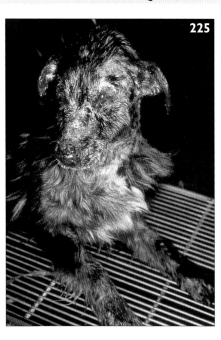

i. What are the differential diagnoses?
ii. The histological findings of the skin biopsy were hydropic degeneration of the basal cells, full thickness necrosis of the epidermis, and minimal inflammation in the dermis. What is the diagnosis?
iii. How should this case be managed, and what is the prognosis?

226 A veterinary dermatologist reported using topical dexamethasone ear drops (1 mg/ml in propylene glycol) for the chronic management of seborrheic otitis externa. How should 60 ml of a dexamethasone otic solution with a concentration of 1 mg/ml of dexamethasone be compounded from dexamethasone 2 mg/ml?

227 What is Norwegian scabies?

225 i. The severe signs of illness limit the differential diagnoses to SLE, severe erythema multiforme, superficial suppurative necrolytic dermatitis, cutaneous lymphoma, drug eruptions, and toxic epidermal necrolysis.

ii. The histological findings are compatible with toxic epidermal necrolysis. The cause of this rare disease is unknown; however, it is usually associated with some other major illness such as a drug reaction or neoplasia. Most cases are idiopathic.

iii. The prognosis for this patient is guarded to poor depending upon identification of the underlying disease. These patients are managed as if they have severe burns: aggressive fluid therapy with attention to electrolyte and colloidal losses, parenteral nutrition, antibiotic therapy for sepsis, and wound management. Pain management is critical for humane reasons.

226 First, calculate the number of mg of dexamethasone needed in 60 ml:

$1 \text{ mg/ml} \times 60 \text{ ml} = 60 \text{ mg}$

Next, calculate how many ml of dexamethasone 2 mg/ml is needed to get the same amount:

$60 \text{ mg} \div 2 \text{ mg/ml} = 30 \text{ ml of dexamethasone at 2 mg/ml}$

Then, calculate the quantity of propylene glycol to add to get a 60 ml solution of dexamethasone 1 mg/ml:

$60 \text{ ml} - 30 \text{ ml} = 30 \text{ ml of propylene glycol}$

Note: the author commonly uses this dexamethasone/propylene glycol otic solution for the treatment of allergic otitis externa and seborrheic otitis in both dogs and cats. This formulation is especially useful in cases where the benefits of glucocorticoids are desired but concurrent application of antimicrobials is not needed or desired.

227 'Norwegian scabies' is the common name for a heavy infestation of scabies mites in a host. This can occur in people or in animals. What is unique about this type of scabies is that the animal is heavily crusted and large numbers of mites are found on skin scraping. It is presumed that the host is immunosuppressed, and this allows large numbers of mites to proliferate. The author has seen one case of Norwegian scabies in a dog with lymphosarcoma. The dog presented with no pruritus and had generalized crusting from the nose to tail, at least 0.5 cm thick. Hundreds of mites were found on skin scraping. Concurrent chemotherapy and lime sulfur were used to treat the dog.

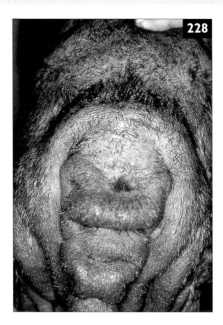

228 The tail base region of a Chinese shar-pei dog is shown (228). The owner complained that the dog is malodorous. It did not take long to localize the source of the odor to the tail region.
i. What is the clinical name for this syndrome, and how is it treated?
ii. What is the pathogenesis of these lesions?
iii. How does 'body odor' occur?

229 Monitoring the various life cycle stages of *Demodex* mites is important in the treatment of demodicosis. What are the various stages of the *Demodex* mite life cycle and how are they identified?

230 What are fipronil, imidacloprid, selamectin, and nitenpyram?

228 i. Intertrigo or fold pyoderma. When folds of skin are in constant apposition, moisture and humidity increase, and bacterial overgrowth results. Fold pyodermas are commonly seen on the face, lips, tail fold area, and vulva. Dogs or cats with anatomical predispositions to fold pyoderma will have chronic bacterial infections of these areas. Surgical correction may or may not be helpful. The success of therapy depends upon whether or not the anatomical defect will redevelop on its own. Daily washings with a mild antibacterial shampoo (e.g. chlorhexidine) are needed to minimize odor, overgrowth, and discomfort. Response to therapy and owner compliance with topical therapy is often hastened by a 21–30 day treatment course of antimicrobials. Concurrent topical therapy with mupirocin ointment may be helpful. Relapses will occur if the client becomes lax with topical therapy. It is important to remember that many of these areas are also colonized by large numbers of *Malassezia* organisms; thus, systemic antifungal and antibacterial therapy may be needed in severe cases.

ii. The primary cause of intertrigo is chronic irritation from repeated friction between two skin folds. Repeated friction occurs in areas where the skin is in constant apposition and also where there is poor air circulation. These two situations result in increased moisture, sebum, glandular secretions (skin, tears, saliva, urine), and an optimal environment for maceration of the skin. Macerated skin is easily over-colonized by bacteria and yeast, that otherwise might not invade the surrounding tissues. These organisms multiply and produce cellular breakdown products that result in odor and increased irritation.

iii. Skin odor is the result of bacterial decomposition of secretions from sebaceous glands, epidermal lipids, and epitrichial and atrichial sweat glands. Epitrichial glands are present on haired skin just below sebaceous glands and open onto the surface via the piliary canal. These glands are largest and most numerous in mucocutaneous junctions, interdigital spaces, and over the dorsal back, and lumbosacral areas. Not surprisingly, this is often where odor concentrates in pets.

Atrichial glands are located only on footpads. Sweat contains unsaturated fatty acids, ammonia constituents, and their volatile salts. Sebum and epidermal lipids on the skin surface are degraded by lipases of Gram-positive bacteria to glycerol and unsaturated fatty acids, which are further metabolized to odorous compounds. It is these by-products that give sebum its antibacterial and antifungal properties. Some of the acids produced by the degradation of these lipids, butyric and caproic acids, are very volatile and emit a cheesy rancid odor. Oral odor may be associated with systemic illnesses such as uremia, diabetes mellitus, or periodontal disease. Malodor associated with periodontal disease is due to the production of volatile sulfur components. Oral odors are most often the result of by-products of bacterial metabolism resulting from bacteria colonization of plaque, gingival sulci, and the dorsal surface of the posterior tongue. Oral odors may also be the result of something the pet has ingested (e.g. fecal material).

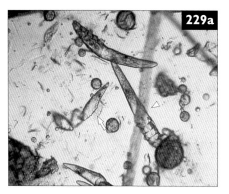
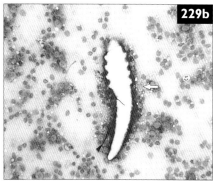

229 Egg, larva, nymph, and adult. Eggs are lemon shaped (229a, arrow), larvae have six legs (229a, arrowhead), and nymphs and adults have eight legs (229b, arrow).

230 These drugs are primarily flea adulticides. Fipronil is a phenylpyrazole that is effective against fleas and ticks. It acts as an antagonist at the flea's GABA receptor and blocks chloride passage. It is a selective neurotoxin and is safe for use in mammals. Imidacloprid is a chloronicotinyl nitroguanidine that binds to nicotinyl receptors on the post-synaptic portion of the insect nerve cell, preventing acetylcholine from binding. This drug has a higher affinity for insect than mammalian receptors and is relatively safe in mammals. It is effective against lice and fleas and newer formulations are also effective against ticks. Selamectin is a semi-synthetic avermectin and is considered to be an endectocide because it is effective against both external and internal parasites (e.g. heartworms, fleas, ear mites, scabies). Nitenpyram is a neonicotinoid and it inhibits nicotinic acetycholine receptors. This product has a rapid onset of action and kills fleas within 15–30 minutes. It does not have any residual activity and is best used for its short acting quick kill in acute flea infestations.

References and recommended reading

Belisto DV (1999). Allergic contact dermatitis. In: *Fitzpatrick's Dermatology in General Practice*, V. IM Freedberg (ed). McGraw-Hill, New York, p.1447.

Bolon B, Calderwood Mays MB, Hall BJ (1990). Characteristics of canine melanomas and comparison of histology and DNA ploidy to their biologic effect. *Veterinary Pathology*, 27: 96–102.

Bregman CL, Hirth RS, Sundberg JP, Chirstensen EF (1987). Cutaneous neoplasms in dogs associated with canine oral papillomavirus vaccine. *Veterinary Pathology*, 24: 477–487.

Breitschwerdt EB, Greene CE (1998). Bartonellosis. In: *Infectious Diseases of the Dog and Cat*, 2nd edn. CE Greene (ed). WB Saunders, Philadelphia, pp. 337–343.

Cannon AG, Affolter VK, Patz J, Gregory CR, Moore PF (2000). Leflunomide for the treatment of canine reactive histiocytosis (abstract) *Veterinary Dermatology*, 11(Suppl.1): 29.

Curtis CF (2001). Evaluation of a commercially available enzyme-linked immunosorbent assay for the diagnosis of canine sarcoptic mange. *Veterinary Record*, 148: 238–239.

DeBoer DJ, Hilliar A (2001). The ACVD task force on canine atopic dermatitis (XVI): laboratory evaluation of dogs with atopic dermatitis with serum based allergy tests. *Veterinary Immunology and Immunopathology*, 81: 277–287.

DeBoer DJ, Marsella R (2001). The ACVD task force on canine atopic dermatitis (XII): the relationship of cutaneous infections to the pathogenesis and clinical course of atopic dermatitis. *Veterinary Immunology and Immunopathology*, 81: 239–249.

Ferguson E (2002). An approach to facial dermatoses. In: *BSAVA Small Animal Dermatology*, 2nd edn. A Foster, C Foil (eds). British Small Animal Veterinary Association, Gloucester UK, pp. 94–103.

Fox LE (2002). Mast cell tumors. In: *Cancer in Dogs and Cats: Medical and Surgical Management*, 2nd edn. WB Morrison (ed). Teton NewMedia, Jackson, pp. 451–460.

Gross TL, Olivry T, Tobin DK (2000). Morphologic and immunologic characterization of a canine isthmus mural folliculitis resembling pseudopelade of humans. *Veterinary Dermatology*, 11: 17–24.

Guillot J, Latié L, Manjula D, Halos L, Chermette R (2001). Evaluation of the dermatophyte test medium Rapid Vet-D. *Veterinary Dermatology*, 12: 123–127.

Halliwell REW (1990). Clinical and immunological aspects of allergic skin diseases. In: *Advances in Veterinary Dermatology*, Vol 1. C Von Tscharner, REW Halliwell (eds). Bailliere Tindall, London UK, pp. 106–111.

Hargis A, Lewis TP (1999). Full-thickness cutaneous burn in black haired skin on the dorsum of a the body of a dalmatian puppy. *Veterinary Dermatology*, 10: 39–42.

Harwick RP (1978). Lesions caused by canine ear mites. *Archives of Veterinary Dermatology*, 114: 130–131.

Headington JT (1993). Telogen effluvium. New concepts and review. *Archives of Dermatology*, 129; 356–363.

Juarbe-Diaz S, Frank L (2002). Acral lick and other compulsive behaviors. In: *BSAVA Small Animal Dermatology*, 2nd edn. A Foster, C Foil (eds). British Small Animal Veterinary Association, Gloucester UK, pp. 116–120.

Kunkle G, Halliwell R (2002). Flea allergy and flea control. In: *BSAVA Small Animal Dermatology*, 2nd edn. A Foster, C Foil (eds). British Small Animal Veterinary Association, Gloucester UK, pp. 137–145.

Linder KE, Kunkle GA, Parker WM, Yager JA (2002). Applications of the skin zenograft mouse model in veterinary dermatology research: modeling canine demodicosis. In: *Advances in Veterinary Dermatology*, Vol 4. KL Thoday, CS Foil, R Bond (eds). Blackwell Publishing, Oxford UK, pp. 76–83.

Lopez RA (1993) Of mites and man. *Journal of the American Veterinary Medical Association*, 203: 606–607.

MacEwan NA (2000). Adherence by *Staphylococcus intermedius* to canine keratinocytes in atopic dermatitis. *Research in Veterinary Science*, 68: 279–283.

Matthews BE (1981). Mechanics of skin penetration of hookworm larvae. *Veterinary Dermatology Newsletter*, 6: 75.

Miller MA, Dunstan RW (1993). Seasonal flank alopecia in boxers and Airedale terriers: 24 cases (1985–1992). *Journal of the American Veterinary Medical Association*, 203: 1567–1572.

Minor RR (1987). Genetic diseases of connective tissue in animals. *Current Problems in Dermatology*, 17: 199.

Moriello KA (2001). Diagnostic techniques for dermatophytosis. *Clinical Techniques in Small Animal Practice*, 16: 219–224.

Noli C (2002). Staphylococcal pyoderma. In: *BSAVA Small Animal Dermatology*, 2nd edn. A Foster, C Foil (eds). British Small Animal Veterinary Association, Gloucester UK, pp. 159–168.

Page N, Paradis M, Lapointe J, Dunstan R (2003). Hereditary nasal parakeratosis in Labrador retrievers. *Veterinary Dermatology*, 14: 103–110.

Paterson S (2002). An approach to focal alopecia in the dog. In: *BSAVA Small Animal Dermatology*, 2nd edn. A Foster, C Foil (eds). British Small Animal Veterinary Association, Gloucester UK, pp. 77–82.

Paterson S, Boydell P, Maxwell M, Whitbread T (1999). Ultrasonographic biomicroscopy to assess changes in the skin after shampoo therapy. In: *Advances in Veterinary Dermatology*, Vol 2. KW Kwochka, T Willemse, C von Tscharner (eds). Butterworth Heinemann, Oxford UK, pp. 523–524.

Power HT, Olivry T, Woo J, Moore PF (1998). Novel feline alopecia areata-like dermatosis: cytotoxic T-lymphocytes target the follicular isthmus. In: *Advances in Veterinary Dermatology*, III. KW Kwochka, T Willemse, C von Tscharner (eds). Butterworth-Heinemann, Boston, p. 538.

Rosser E, Dunstan RW (1998). Sporotrichosis. In: *Infectious Diseases of the Dog and Cat*, 2nd edn. CE Greene (ed). WB Saunders, Philadelphia, pp. 399–402.

Saridomichelakis MN (1999). Sensitization to house dust mites in cats with *Otodectes cynotis* infestation. *Veterinary Dermatology*, 10: 89–94.

Scott DW (2002). An approach to diseases of claws and claw folds. In: *BSAVA Small Animal Dermatology*, 2nd edn. A Foster, C Foil (eds). British Small Animal Veterinary Association, Gloucester UK, pp. 116–120.

Scott DW, Miller WH, Griffin CE (2001a). Parasitic skin diseases. In: *Muller & Kirk's Small Animal Dermatology*, 6th edn. WB Saunders, Philadelphia, pp. 423–515.

Scott DW, Miller WH, Griffin CE (2001b). Bacterial skin diseases. In: *Muller & Kirk's Small Animal Dermatology*, 6th edn. WB Saunders, Philadelphia, pp. 274–335.

Scott DW, Miller WH, Griffin CE (2001c). Environmental skin diseases. In: *Muller & Kirk's Small Animal Dermatology*, 6th edn. WB Saunders, Philadelphia, pp. 1073–1109.

Scott DW, Miller WH, Griffin CE (2001d). Keratinization defects. In: *Muller & Kirk's Small Animal Dermatology*, 6th edn. WB Saunders, Philadelphia, pp. 1073–1109.

Scott DW, Miller WH, Griffin CE (2001e). Congenital and hereditary defects. In: *Muller & Kirk's Small Animal Dermatology*, 6th edn. WB Saunders, Philadelphia, p. 979.

Scott DW, Miller WH, Griffin CE (2001f). Congenital and hereditary defects. In: *Muller & Kirk's Small Animal Dermatology*, 6th edn. WB Saunders, Philadelphia, p. 996.

Scott DW, Miller WH, Griffin CE (2001g). Acquired alopecias. In: *Muller & Kirk's Small Animal Dermatology*, 6th edn. WB Saunders, Philadelphia, pp. 893–894.

Scott DW, Miller WH, Griffin CE (2001h). Acquired alopecias. In: *Muller & Kirk's Small Animal Dermatology*, 6th edn. WB Saunders, Philadelphia, pp. 887–893.

Scott DW, Miller WH, Griffin CE (2001i). Immune-mediated disorders. In: *Muller & Kirk's Small Animal Dermatology*, 6th edn. WB Saunders, Philadelphia, pp. 667–779.

Scott DW, Miller WH, Griffin CE (2001j), Pigmentary abnormalities. In: *Muller & Kirk's Small Animal Dermatology*, 6th edn. WB Saunders, Philadelphia, pp. 1018–1019.

Shearer D, Dobson J (2002). An approach to nodules and draining sinuses In: *BSAVA Small Animal Dermatology*, 2nd edn. A Foster, C Foil (eds). British Small Animal Veterinary Association, Gloucester UK, pp. 55–65.

Slappendel RJ, Ferrer L (1998). Leishmaniasis. In: *Infectious Diseases of the Dog and Cat*, 2nd edn. CE Greene (ed). WB Saunders, Philadelphia, pp. 451–458.

Smith JD, Goette DK, Odom RB (1976). Larva currens: cutaneous strongyloidiasis. *Archives of Dermatology*, **1121**: 161–163.

Tapp RA, Roy AF, Corstvet RE, Wilson VL (2001). Differential selection of *Bartonella* species and strains in cat scratch disease by polymerase chain reaction amplification of 16S ribosomal RNA gene. *Journal of Veterinary Diagnostic Investigation*, **13**(3): 219–229.

Thamm DH, Vail DM (2001). Mast cell tumors. In: *Small Animal Clinical Oncology*, 3rd edn. SJ Withrow, EG MacEwen (eds). WB Saunders, Philadelphia, pp. 261–282.

Thomas RC, Fox LE (2002). Tumors of the skin and subcutis. In: *Cancer in Dogs and Cats: Medical and Surgical Management*, 2nd edn. WB Morrison (ed). Teton NewMedia, Jackson, pp. 469–488.

Turin L, Riva F, Galbiati G, Cainelli T (2000). Fast, simple, and high sensitive double-rounded polymerase chain reaction assay to detect medically relevant fungi in dermatological specimens. *European Journal of Clinical Investigation*, **30**(6): 511–518.

Turner JA (1962). Human dipylidiasis (dog tapeworm infection) in the United States. *Journal of Pediatrics*, **61**: 763–768.

Vail DM, Withrow SJ (2001). Tumors of the skin and subcutaneous tissues. In: *Small Animal Clinical Oncology*, 3rd edn. SJ Withrow, EG MacEwen (eds). WB Saunders, Philadelphia, pp. 233–260.

Walder EJ, Hargis AM (2002). Chronic moderate heat dermatitis (erythema ab igne) in five dogs, three cats, and one silvered langur. *Veterinary Dermatology*, **13**: 283–292.

Zhang X, Andrews JH (1993). Evidence for the growth of *Sporothrix schenkii* on dead but not on living sphagnum moss. *Mycopathalogia*, **123**: 87–94.

Znajda NR, Grooters AM, Marsella R (2002). PCR-based detection of *Pythium* and *Lagenidium* DNA in frozen and ethanol-fixed animal tissues. *Veterinary Dermatology*, **13**: 187–194.

Index

Index

Index